Praise f or Son Down, Son Up

"I was there at the Celebrate Recovery program at Cokesbury Church in Knoxville, Tennessee, when Brenda, and eventually Jamie and Matthew, walked through the doors and into a new life. I was there because I was also a recovering addict and, at that point, a volunteer working in the program. In her book, Brenda describes the hell her son went through as he traveled through his addiction. She describes the hell all addicts go through. She describes the hell I went through. And now, at last, she has described her own hell and that of all parents of addicts.

"Over the years since then, and as I have continued working to help others escape the chains of addiction as I had, I have heard Brenda's words spoken by so many parents. Although I'm sure Brenda felt unique in her battle against the "Beast," she faced the same enemy that countless other mothers and fathers faced then and are facing today. Her words will bring the light of hope into those parents' dark worlds. Her words will help those parents wage war against the addiction that is killing their children. Her words will show those parents a way out of the hell they live in.

"Every story of addiction has an ending. Some of those endings are tragic. But, your story of addiction doesn't have to end in tragedy if you follow the steps that Brenda followed. Love your addict. Stop enabling your addict. Get help in a Christ-centered recovery program. At the end of this book, Brenda explains what she hoped to accomplish in writing it. She wanted to give parents hope that their child could overcome addiction. She wanted to let them know that they didn't cause the addiction. And finally, she wanted to draw attention to the fact that good people can be addicts. She accomplished all three in an open, honest telling of her own story that will give you strength to continue your own battle with the Beast."

—Jerry Smith,
Grateful recovering addict saved by grace
Founder of Havenwood, Chairman of the Board for
Recovery At Ringgold, part of the Recovery At
Cokesbury Network

"It takes only a few pages of *Son Down, Son Up* to grasp the riveting detail of a mother's courageous love for a son as she tracks him into the abysses of the unfathomable darkness of addictive insanity. Brenda Seals provides us with a rare glimpse of a parent's heartbreaking terror and ghastly surprise in finding her child in the diabolical grip of The Beast. At the brink of hopelessness, the Grace of God brings special friends and faith-based programs of recovery into Brenda's life that begins to show her that The Beast is no match for the unconditional love of a mother and her Heavenly Father. This is not just a book for mothers, but for any parent and family concerned – as they should be – for children growing up in an addictive-saturated society. There is a Beast who seeks to devour; but we worship a God who has already defeated the Beast. God will give you the grace – as He did to Brenda – to fight your battles for yourself, your children, family, community and world."

—Dr. Gil Smith, retired Celebrate Recovery Director

"What an accurate description of a mother of an addict. It gives HOPE to mothers like me who are still praying for their children battling The Beast. Brenda's story of faith has blessed me, and I praise God for Matthew's recovery!"

—Cyndy, mother of an active addict

"Nothing stronger than a Mother's love! By sharing her pain and mistakes made along the way, Brenda gives hope and healing to other families struggling with a loved one in the grips of active addiction. The entire families' individual perspectives were captured in a way that truly drives home the concept of addiction affecting the entire family. Brenda, Kudos to you and your family for putting such a wonderful book together. I've not seen one where everyone in the family shared their perspective. I always emphasize that this is a family disease and all are affected. This certainly spoke to that very thing, but you sure carried the load. As mothers, we do these things and tend to keep going when we are literally ready to fall apart. You should be so very proud of yourself for having the courage to share your journey with others. So many families who have lost someone share their story, but few who have someone in recovery take the time to share the fact that there is HOPE. Thank you again for allowing me the amazing honor of reading your incredible journey! So happy for all of you that Matthew is doing so well."

—Karen Pershing, MPH, CPS II,
Metro Drug Coalition Executive Director

"Wow! So much truth is now available for all the lost parents of addicts. As a pastor over a Celebrate Recovery, I get twice the number of calls from parents than I do from those struggling. Sadly, most parents do not follow my advice. Now I can hand them this book and pray they follow Brenda's. Thank you Brenda for being honest, available and vulnerable. I pray the process of writing this book equals the blessing I received by reading it. God bless you."

—Rev. John Gargis

"As a therapist, I have heard many heartbreaking stories of so many parents. Ms. Seals shares her difficult journey of loving her son and learning to love without enabling his disease of addiction. She also recognized her need to "fix" him and how that trait was adding to the problems. The book is insightful, compassionate, brave, and educational. All of us can benefit and gain hope from this family."

—Vicky McDaniel, LPC, Clinical Director, Cokesbury Counseling Center

"We are an ordinary husband and wife who began a journey of drug addiction involving our son over five years ago. Our experiences mirror much of Brenda's. Hope is a theme in Brenda's storyline and must become part of your daily life. Spend time with the 32 questions listed at the end of the book. Read this outstanding documentary with an understanding that this story could become you or is you today."

—Al & Jackie North, Celebrate Recovery Tennessee State Reps

Son Down, Son Up

Drug addicts are not good people
So don't try to tell me
That they are worth saving
Because we all know
They are worthless, awful people
And nothing will make me think
They deserve to be loved
Realizing they are someone's child and
That the pain might be too hard to bear
Makes matters worse, and just
Because we say it could happen to anyone
We have to ask, why do we care?

—Brenda Seals

Now, read the poem again, but from the bottom up.

Son Down, Son Up

Son Down, Son Up

How One Mother
Battled Her Son's Addiction,
Found Hope, and Survived

Brenda Seals

Crippled Beagle Publishing

Scripture quotations are from The ESV® Bible (The Holy Bible, English Standard Version®), copyright © 2001 by Crossway, a publishing ministry of Good News Publishers. Used by permission. All rights reserved.

Scriptures taken from the Holy Bible, New International Version®, NIV®. Copyright © 1973, 1978, 1984, 2011 by Biblica, Inc.™ Used by permission of Zondervan. All rights reserved worldwide. www.zondervan.com The "NIV" and "New International Version" are trademarks registered in the United States Patent and Trademark Office by Biblica, Inc.™

Crippled Beagle Publishing
Knoxville, Tennessee
dyer.cbpublishing@gmail.com

Cover and book design by Jody Dyer
Cover photo taken by Jamie Seals

ISBN 978-1-970037-16-6

Dedicated to my husband Jim and my children Matthew, Courtney, and Kimberly. Without your support and love, I could never have told my story through this book.

My Son Is An Opioid Addict

I TELL MYSELF, "He doesn't do heroin now. He is not an addict anymore." I'm not sure what the proper term is. *Recovered? Recovering?* When you say someone is an alcoholic or a drug addict, you use the present tense. Matthew is now clean, but for many years my life was a living hell. I like to think of Matthew as a recovered addict, but to be truthful, he's still recovering. All of Matthew's loved ones are still recovering.

The term *drug addict* sounds so dirty. Isn't it ironic that the opposite of dirty is *clean*, and *clean* is used to describe addicts who are not using? Even though my son's addiction put our family through absolute turmoil, I don't have the heart to call my son addict. I could, however, call my dad an alcoholic until the day he died. Maybe that is because he never tried to get well.

Why the stigma for a drug addict? A diabetic is always a diabetic. He or she can change his or her lifestyle and attempt to manage the disease, but that person will always be diabetic.

There's no shame attached. Someone with diabetes who continues bad eating habits or hesitates to exercise is rarely openly ridiculed.

Former United States Surgeon General Vivek Murthy stated addiction is a chronic disease of the brain. He also stated that for far too long people have thought about addiction as a character flaw or a moral failing. As long as people feel that way, it will impede and slow down the war on drugs. Investing money into treatment and recovery is urgently needed. The war on drugs is not going away. It is getting worse.

During the horror of Matthew's heroin addiction, I found myself asking, "Why my son?" "Why my family?" "Why *me*?"

I am just one mom, but I am not alone. Drug addiction is an epidemic. I have heard the same story hundreds of times from other suffering parents. We use the same words. Our children's names are different, we live in different cities and states, but we share the same painful story. The child can be the class president, the star football player, an All-American cheerleader, an honor student, or a good Christian, yet the stories are the same.

The Beast does not discriminate.

The Beast possesses the child.

You miss the signs. You think that The Beast will never come knocking on your door, that you are immune, that you are safe, but The Beast will do whatever it takes to slide, sneak, or crash into your life.

The Beast takes the child's soul. Then it takes yours. Then it takes both of you down—down into the darkest place you can imagine. It takes you to a place you never thought you would be, a place so dark that the addict sees no way out. The parent sees no way out. You worry where your child is. Is he alone? Is he in some dark room, surrounded by other addicts who don't care about him? Is he on the street? Is he in a filthy building? Is he hungry? Is he even alive?

When your child is addicted to drugs, you endure terrible situations weekly, daily, and moment by moment. There is no escape from worry. You cry, beg, plead, and threaten, but it does no good. Such futile attempts to persuade the addict only make you feel sadder and weaker. A mother cannot *make* an addict stop using drugs. There is no "Just say no" once addiction has taken hold of your child. You hope the trauma will end, and you know it can end in tragedy. You suffer deep painful heartache; you can't comprehend that any pain could be as severe.

When your children are young, you know what to do when they are sick and hurting. When they are older and using drugs, you are lost. You feel alone. You are ashamed, so you don't tell any of your friends, your coworkers, even your spouse. Guilt and anxiety become your constant companions.

There is tremendous stigma attached to addiction and the addicted; fear of the stigma itself often deters addicts from seeking help. Addiction is <u>common</u>. You probably know someone who is addicted.

Once hooked, addiction is not a choice. Yes, whether to try drugs in the first place is a choice, but once the chemical is in the body, it changes the structure of the brain, which, over time, drastically alters a person's decision-making. At that point addiction supersedes family, socio-economic status, willpower, character, morality, intelligence, and faith.

Addiction is a powerful progressive disease; without treatment it only gets worse. Addiction affects the addict's entire family. Everyone is drawn in and hurt by the lies and manipulation. There can also be serious financial consequences when a family is supporting an addict. Parents may lose everything, even their savings and their homes. Some file bankruptcy. If parents run out of or stop giving the addict money, The Beast steers the addict toward grandparents, friends, coworkers, and others. The Beast sucks in people close to the addict and joyfully watches them wallow in the nightmare. It wants to take everyone down.

During the worst years of my son's addiction, I searched bookstores for stories written by parents of addicts. I searched for hope. I became frustrated by many of the book descriptions because they all appeared dreadful. I wanted at least one book that offered promise—one book in which the addict got well and clean and was still well and clean years later. I never found that book.

I desired the kind of hope that is life-changing—hope that would dwell in my soul and enable me to face demons. I needed the kind of hope that would allow me to sleep without worrying about Matthew and his decisions—decisions that could cost him his life. I needed the kind of hope that allowed me to believe he would survive.

That kind of hope can be found only in the spiritual realm. That hope is found only in the presence of Jesus Christ.

Wishing may lead to frustration and depression. Hoping is *believing* that something WILL happen.

Wishes are something *we* want.

Hope is about what *God* wants.

Are you wishing or hoping?

For countless nights I went to bed wishing Matthew would stop using drugs and wishing I could get him to stop. Only when my wishes evolved into hopes, and I trusted Jesus to take control did lives begin to change.

Years ago, I felt called to write a book about finding hope in the pit of addiction. I knew there would be healing in telling my story, but I struggled for years to write that story. I grieved that there was even a need for the telling of that kind of story. Part of me didn't want to bring up the ugly past. Part of me wanted to forget and move on. I was worried that my son wouldn't want me to expose his past. God placed sign after sign in my path to usher me toward writing my story. I came up with excuse after excuse and reason after reason why I couldn't write, but everywhere I turned, the compelling signs to go forward were right in front of me. Friend after friend said, "You have to write a book and tell your story." One gave me the name of a publisher; I kept it for a bit but eventually threw it away. One day I pulled up social media on my computer and an ad for a book writing workshop came up. I walked into a bookstore once and the first book cover I spotted read, "Do you have a story to tell?" I went to hear a speaker and when I bought her book, she signed my copy and wrote, "Listen to God's whisper to you, and act on it." I felt compelled to write the book that I had needed because I knew millions of parents were in a living hell. There are mothers and fathers who pray without ceasing for their children. There are parents who cry themselves to sleep at night only to wake up and immediately wonder where their children are and if they are still alive. I wrote this book for them. I certainly don't have all the answers, but I know what worked for me.

I survived a nightmare, a nightmare that is especially hard for mothers. But the nightmare also exists for fathers, sisters, brothers, relatives, spouses, children, and friends of addicts. I am not a psychologist, psychiatrist, or addiction specialist. I have no formal training, but I lived through the nightmare of a child with an addiction.

When I sat down to write, my goal was to reach the largest number of people that I could. I wondered whether or not to include a religious context. I was afraid that some people would be turned off by the mention of God, but in my heart, I knew that God was with me every step of the way and that He paved the road for both my healing and Matthew's recovery.

If there is one thing I would like for people to take away from my story, it is HOPE. Hope is what we have to hold on to during a loved one's addiction. When Matthew was deep in the bowels of Hell, I looked for and needed hope. I went searching high and low for one book that had a successful ending with the addict clean. I could not find one. Not. One. Book. I realize there is not always a good outcome for everyone battling an addiction. My heart goes out to those who grieve. My story is one of hope and proof that it is possible for an addict to get clean and well. I am now willing—through God's mercy and grace—to offer my experience as a gift of hope to let others know you can survive this and so can your loved ones. God never gave up on Matthew, and he hasn't given up on me. This is my story.

Childhood Survival

MY FAMILY WAS MIDDLE-CLASS and appeared to be normal. It wasn't. We kept secrets. My father was an alcoholic who abused my mother, and no one knew. He was always an alcoholic, but the abuse got worse after he was in an accident that caused him to become disabled. When he could no longer work, I guess he lost what little self-esteem and self-worth he had. He would start drinking first thing in the morning. By nighttime he would be totally drunk. He took all of his anger out on my mother. He screamed at her, called her names, and hit her. It didn't take much for him to get mad enough to start yelling, and it didn't take long for him to hit her. She could accidentally block his view of the TV, and he would get mad enough to start yelling and hitting her or threatening to hit her.

I am surprised that Christmas is my favorite holiday because our Christmases were always ruined by alcohol. As my brothers and I opened our presents, we held our breath because we never knew what would set our father off. When

I was little, I begged my mother not to say anything that would cause my father to get angry. She kept quiet, but he still found reasons to hit her. She gave up. I suppose she had had enough. She started talking back to him and making him angrier. Nothing helped. He abused her emotionally or physically whether she submitted or rebelled.

The abuse got so severe and so frequent that I never wanted to be away from home. Once I went to spend the night with my cousin, but when bedtime came I got scared. I was scared of my mother being home alone with him. I told my uncle I was homesick and wanted to go home, but I was really just afraid my father would kill my mother while I was gone. My oldest brother had moved out and was living with my grandmother, and my next oldest brother had joined the Army. I was left to fend for and protect my mother and younger brother. I guess you could say (or at least I felt) that I was the only person who could "fix" the problem. It was an incomprehensible burden. During my father's rages I latched on to him and cried and begged him not to hit my mother. My tactic worked every time. My father never laid a hand on me. After his outbursts, he went to bed and slept off his drunkenness.

When he woke up the next morning, he always acted like nothing had happened. My father was also manipulative. He would walk me over to a calendar on the wall and draw a big red circle around a date. The date was usually one or two weeks out, and he would tell me that he was going to stop drinking on that day. The day always came and went, but he never stopped. My mother lived a hell on earth, and I lived my own hell right beside her. My mother is one of the finest

Christian women I know. In her generation and culture, divorce was unthinkable. In those times, people rarely divorced. They stayed stuck in bad situations. She did the best she could to make our house a home and do what she thought was right. She is a strong woman who tolerated a lot more than I ever would have endured. I have always admired her efforts to keep our family together.

My father was one of thirteen children. One died as a baby. Another died extremely young. A third sibling died two weeks after getting married. He was killed in a parking lot when a gunman mistook him for someone else. Of the remaining ten, five became alcoholics. There was an obvious predisposition toward addiction in his family.

My father died of lung cancer three weeks after being diagnosed. He never stopped drinking. After he died, I was angry at him for a very long time. It wasn't until I went to a Bible study at my church that I was finally able to forgive him. I remember asking the group, "How do you forgive someone who never asks for forgiveness?" They explained that I had to forgive him for my own health and peace of mind. I didn't really understand it at the time, but I tried. Now, many years later, I realize that if I am to go on with my life, I cannot hold on to anger.

On his deathbed my father tried to whisper something to me. When I got close to him, all he could do was cry. He tried to open his mouth to speak, but nothing came out. I like to think he was going to say he was sorry.

His side of the family thought he was wonderful because he was always giving money to my cousins and buying drinks and food for everyone. Years later they told me they thought he was rich. They didn't know that he spent money on them and on alcohol but gave very little to my mother to support us.

We never spoke about his drinking or abuse outside our immediate family. My friends didn't know, and other family members had no idea what our lives were really like. In public we were a "normal" family. At home, we were a mess. I was scared, lonely, and embarrassed. Out of fear and shame, I learned as a child how to keep enormous secrets.

Leaving Home

I FINALLY HAD THE COURAGE TO MOVE OUT on my own after I graduated from high school and turned eighteen. I couldn't live in that chaotic house anymore. I couldn't stand all the turmoil. There was so much drama. Numerous times I begged my mother to leave, but she always said, "Half a home is better than no home at all." To this day, I'm not sure what she meant; I guess she thought living in a home with two parents, regardless of how awful life was, was better than struggling with a single mother in a tiny apartment. I felt guilty for leaving home, but I did it anyway. My mother needed to save herself.

I wanted to go to college, but in order to live independently, I had to work. I got a full-time job and moved into a one-bedroom apartment. I was in love with my high school sweetheart. He was a great guy, but that didn't work out. I started dating all over again.

Many girls are lucky that they can dream of marrying men just like their fathers. While I loved my father, and I know he loved me, I did not want to marry anyone like him. I did not want to marry someone who would ever hit me or be mentally or emotionally abusive. A couple of years after I moved out on my own, my cousin introduced me to a cute guy she knew. We dated, and two years later we got married.

Motherhood

WHEN I FOUND OUT I WAS PREGNANT, I was ecstatic. I couldn't wait to be a mother. One of my good friends at work was also expecting. We ate lunch together every day just so we could compare our pregnancies: how we felt, (I felt great, she was tired), eating habits (I liked sweet things, she didn't), weight gain (I gained very little and she gained about 40 pounds), and due dates. I found out I was having a boy pretty early on and, of course, started buying everything blue. Since I had two older brothers and one younger brother, I felt confident in my ability to raise a boy.

Back then, I was a competitive softball player. I did not want to give up softball when I was pregnant, so I actually did some pretty dumb stunts. I slid into second base when I was about three months pregnant and my oldest brother, who was the coach, came onto the field and jerked me out of the game and made me sit on the bench. He yelled at me all the way to the dugout. I wasn't happy with him then, but now I totally understand why he did it.

When I was eight months pregnant I was practicing softball when I felt like something wasn't right. I started having side pains and back pain. First, I thought I might have pulled a muscle. I called my doctor and he told me he didn't think I was in labor because he had just seen me two days before, and I wasn't really even dilated. He told me to come on in and he would examine me. When I got there, he told me I actually was in labor and to immediately go across the street to the hospital. Maybe I shouldn't have been running around on that ball field.

I was in labor almost 30 hours. My baby was breech, which meant he was born bottom first. The doctor tried turning him, but he wouldn't budge. Epidurals wouldn't take. I cried and pleaded for pain relief. When I had contractions, the monitor would peak and stay at the peak for abnormally long intervals, which proved I was in severe pain and my baby was under stress. The physician sent me for X-rays to see if I could actually deliver the baby in his breech position. Today, obstetricians won't even consider it. I blacked out from the pain while going up to X-rays, and again when the nurses brought me down to my labor room. They started another epidural and then I waited and waited and waited. Finally, my son was born!

He was early by at least three weeks, but he was adorable. Aren't they all? He had a head full of dark hair and actually had his first haircut when he was six *weeks* old. Everyone kept looking at him and remarking that "she" was so cute because his hair was so long, so I decided to get it cut. He had enough hair for two or three babies.

When Matthew was born, I didn't even have a name picked out for him. You would think, since I was told he was going to be a boy, I would have chosen a name. I didn't really trust the tests and was working so hard to pay bills that I had little time to think. I was too frantic to make big decisions as I navigated a tough marriage and anticipated motherhood. As I lay in the hospital, I watched my favorite TV show, "Dynasty." The cutest guy on there was Matthew Blaisdel. So, I named my handsome son *Matthew*.

Divorce

WHEN MATTHEW WAS STILL A BABY, being married to my husband was emotionally and physically fatiguing. He was not the man I thought he was. Out of respect for Matthew, I won't elaborate. I will simply say that I was shocked and devastated. Matthew was an infant, but there was no need to prolong the inevitable. I had lived with secrets and with parents who shouldn't have stayed together. I was determined to protect Matthew's innocence and childhood, and I refused to raise Matthew in a home with an unhealthy marriage. When I told my mother I was divorcing and why, she—who had endured years of beatings from my father—looked at me and asked, "What did you do to make this happen?" Her thinking was skewed. I thought, *Really, mother?* I was anxious but determined to be a good mother and raise my son in a healthy environment.

We divorced, and I did my best to raise Matthew on my own. I, of course, had to work, so I put Matthew in a private home for care. He stayed there when he was a baby, and when he was two I moved him to daycare. I didn't date much while he was an infant, but I did manage to have fun with friends on occasional weekends. My mother watched Matthew for me when I would go out. I had two relationships that were serious, each lasted about one year. One of the men was also recently divorced, but he had three very small children, and, even though he was a great guy, I knew it wasn't going to work out. Four young children together would make things too difficult. The other man was ten years older than I was. I stopped seeing him because another woman showed up on his doorstep the same night I did. She said he had invited her to come over. When I questioned her, she left to call him at a phone booth (this was before cell phones) while I stayed on the front porch. While she was gone, he let me in and promised that he had not invited her. She came back to the house and he talked to her outside for about 30 minutes. I thought, *so why not open the door and confront her so I can hear?* What do you say in 30 minutes? When she left, I left, too. I never went back.

A Mind Of His Own

FROM THE TIME MATTHEW was old enough to do things for himself, that's what he did. Long before he started kindergarten, he made his own bed and got himself dressed every morning. As soon as he started school, *every* morning he preheated the oven to the right temperature, got dressed, went back to the kitchen, opened a can of biscuits, placed them on a cookie sheet, and put them in the oven. He set the timer and finished getting dressed. He returned to the kitchen, got the biscuits out of the oven, buttered them, and ate them—all while I got ready for work.

Matthew innately understood the load I carried. He was so good about helping me around the house. He was a little man. After the dishwasher finished a cycle, Matthew emptied it. He got a chair from the kitchen table and put away the dishes in the upper cabinets. Every opportunity he got, he told me that he would always take care of me. Talk about melting my heart! The kid had me at "Mom."

Matthew was very conscious that we were a one-income family and that I was trying very hard to make ends meet with a house note, a car note, and a small child to raise. He never asked for anything we couldn't afford. I'm still amazed when I think about how responsible and grown up he acted at such a young age.

In third grade, Matthew became a "latchkey" child. We lived only one block from the school, so every afternoon he walked home, unlocked the back door, and called me at work to let me know he was home. He stayed in the house and didn't open the door for anyone. He knew not to do anything but watch TV, and I completely trusted him.

If I didn't take Matthew to church, my mother did. Any time I went out on a Saturday night to relax with friends, she had Matthew stay overnight with her. My mother made sure Matthew was in church on those Sunday mornings. My father was also there but was able to control his anger and behavior when Matthew was around him. My father was good to Matthew.

I believe it is important for children to grow up in church. They need to hear Bible stories and play with other children who are growing up with good principles. They need to learn the stories of Jesus and trust the certainty of God. They must learn to pray. They should hear over and over that God loves them and is there, no matter their circumstances. They must understand mercy and grace. They need to know they can't do anything bad enough that God won't forgive them. What in the world do children in crisis do if they don't trust God? To whom do they turn when family fails them?

It was an emotionally difficult season for me while Matthew was under seven because I wanted to do everything right. I strived to raise him to know Jesus. We said prayers every evening. I thanked God aloud for Matthew to hear. I intended to take him to church regularly but was often too exhausted. Thankfully, when I fell short, my mother was on it. She is one of the godliest women I know. Now 91, she has tithed every week of her adult life. Mom even tithed during my childhood when she worried if we would have money for our needs. To this day, my husband and I tithe at our church. I feel it is important because it is what God asks us to do. Churches need funding to stay open and spread the word of Christ through ministry programs. I call my mother my prayer warrior. I sometimes wonder if she has a direct line to God. I suppose that's how she survived her marriage and still had love for my father.

Jim

I MET JIM when a coworker invited me to a Christmas party. The evening of the party, rain was pouring down. On the way there, I changed my mind and decided not to go because it was such a nasty evening. I actually pulled into a driveway to turn around and go back home. Then I decided that I had nothing else to do, so I might as well go. I pulled out of the driveway and headed toward the party. When I got to the house, it was packed with people I didn't know. As a matter of fact, I didn't know a single person at the party except the coworker who'd invited me. He had invited me because he wanted to introduce to me to a particular friend of his. Someone led me to the dining room table where all of the food was, so I stood there for a few minutes and then this man named Jim introduced himself to me. We talked for quite some time, and then he invited me to go to another party. I never did see the guy I worked with, nor did I meet the guy he planned to introduce to me. I went with Jim to his other party. I guess you could say it was fate that turned me around in that driveway on a rainy December night.

Jim and I started dating. He had recently finished medical school and was working on his internship, so he was at the hospital most of the time. Matthew and I would go to the hospital to eat dinner with Jim and keep him company when he was on call. Jim often took Matthew to the hospital call room and let him play at the pool table. When Jim wasn't working, he would spend time at our house.

I was adept at single-parenting, and Matthew was independent and easy, but I do think Jim brought a lot of stability to Matthew's life. After my divorce, my ex-husband told me he would not be Matthew's babysitter. I guess he thought that would stop me from going out with friends or dating. Matthew's father rarely saw Matthew, and Jim was a consistent, kind presence.

There was a time, after Jim and I had dated for about two and a half years that we broke up for about six weeks. Jim was feeling internal pressure to either go forward with our relationship or to end it so I could move on. During the time we were apart, Matthew frequently came home from school with drawings of his "family"—Matthew, Jim, and me. It didn't matter what the drawing was about; it always framed the three of us together. Matthew often asked me to send the pictures to Jim. I said I would, but I kept them at home because I wasn't in touch with Jim. After about five weeks, I called Jim and told him I needed to see him. I showed him Matthew's stack of drawings. I said, "I am doing fine, but apparently Matthew isn't."

I felt Jim owed it to Matthew to tell him what was going on. When I started to leave, Jim grabbed my hand and asked me to wait. He later told me that at that very moment he knew he wanted to marry me. I had no idea. After he saw those colorings that Matthew had drawn and I turned to leave, he realized he was in too deep to let either of us go. Jim asked if I would go out with him the next weekend. I wasn't really sure where he and I were headed, but I agreed to go. Our courtship resumed, and six months later Jim proposed. Matthew was happy. So was I! We were married within three months of becoming engaged.

When Matthew was eight, we moved from Memphis, Tennessee, to Knoxville, Tennessee. After we moved to Knoxville, as far as I know, Matthew's father saw him only one time.

All-American Boy

I CAN'T TELL YOU THE NUMBER OF TIMES I have listened to people talk about their perfect children or grandchildren. Their children are by far the brightest cutest children on earth. I understand. I raised three bright, cute children!

Matthew excelled in academics and sports. When he was young, Matthew loved to read and be read to. He would sit for hours with books piled around him or in my lap (or my mother's lap) for story time. Matthew was always on the elementary school honor roll, and teachers loved him.

When Matthew was nine, my first daughter was born. Matthew was excited to be a big brother and really didn't mind that his baby sibling was a girl. I wanted to name her Brittney, but Matthew had a crush on a girl named Courtney in his fourth-grade class. He said we could name our baby Brittney but he would call her Courtney. I realized he was sincere and engaged, so *Brittney* was out and *Courtney* was in!

Matthew loved having a little sister, and he was good to her. Even though they were nine years apart, Matthew included Courtney. Often, she would be right in the middle of his pack of friends. When Matthew left to go to school in the mornings, he kissed her goodbye. Then she stood on the porch and waved until he was out of sight. They were always close. Our second daughter Kimberly came along three years later. Matthew was a proud big brother again, but he was twelve by the time Kimberly was born. A twelve-year-old boy hanging out with an infant was a bit of a stretch, but Kimberly is the funny one in the family, and he laughed at her hilarious stunts and sayings. When he left home at eighteen to go to college, Courtney was nine and Kimberly was six.

Fixing Failure

MATTHEW STARTED PLAYING SPORTS at around five or six years old. His first athletic venture was baseball. He played pitcher and shortstop. On offense he was the clean-up batter. It made sense, genetically speaking. Matthew comes from a long line of baseball players. My oldest brother was asked to sign out of high school by the St. Louis Cardinals. This was before the draft. Scouts came and watched him play and came to my parents' house to sign him. Unfortunately for him, he was seventeen and needed my parents' written permission for him to go. My parents said he needed a college degree and *made* him go to college. He is 71 and still plays softball and baseball in a 50 and older group. Not long ago, he was inducted into the Memphis Amateur Sports Hall of Fame. My middle brother was a state champion in baseball, while my younger brother also excelled on the diamond. Even my mother played slow pitch softball well into her 50's, and I played fast pitch and slow pitch softball for seventeen years. Matthew tried all of the sports, including soccer and football, but when he picked up a basketball for the first time, he found his sport. He loved the game, and he excelled at it. For seven straight years, no matter which team he was on, he was recognized as the Most Valuable Player (MVP).

I remember when a referee at one of the basketball games walked over to Matthew during a timeout and told him he needed to let the other kids on his team shoot the ball. When Matthew came off the court, his coach asked him what the referee had said. Matthew's coach was furious. He walked out and said something (who knows what) to the referee, and then proceeded to tell Matthew to shoot the ball every time he got it. One of his coaches, at the awards ceremony, gave Matthew his award last. Again, he was the MVP. His coach said, "One day I'm going to be watching a college basketball game, and I am going to hear this young man's name called out, and I'm going to proudly boast that I coached him when he was a kid." We owned everything that Michael Jordan ever sold. Matthew was a superstar—the next Michael Jordan—at least in my eyes!

That all changed when Matthew tried out for his middle school basketball team. He got cut. He was shocked and devastated. We all were. For days, he was very quiet. I said I was going to speak with the coach. He asked me not to because he would be embarrassed, and I would make things worse. I promised I wouldn't, but being the *good* mother I am, I called the school the next day and asked to speak to the coach. I gently asked him what Matthew needed to work on because he planned to try out for the team the next year. He told me that Matthew was an excellent player, better than most of the kids on the team, but while Matthew was a great individual player, he needed a team full of good team players. What? Wasn't Matthew what coaches want and need? A great player? I politely asked him, "Isn't that what good coaches do? Develop great individual players to be great team players?" I told him I really hoped Matthew would still try out the next year. He told me to encourage Matthew to do that. Matthew didn't pick up a basketball for a long time. He neither played with kids in the neighborhood nor played on any youth league teams. I think Matthew was extremely disappointed. There was nothing I could do for him. Jim felt badly for Matthew; he encouraged him to keep playing and to try out again the next year. When the time came, I pleaded with Matthew to go out for the team again, but he would have no part of it. Failure was not something Matthew was used to, especially in sports. Though he quit playing basketball for a long time, no other behaviors changed. We were thankful that his grades and friends remained the same.

Socially Acceptable

MATTHEW WAS A LIKABLE KID. I often joked that he was the neighborhood social director because all of the kids called him to see what everyone was doing. He was certainly one of the "cool kids" in high school. All his friends liked to hang out at our house. Their rowdiest activity (that I knew about) was yard rolling—that's a term for throwing toilet paper all over someone's house and lawn. For them, the target was usually one of the boys' girl crushes. They would run off with bags and bags of toilet paper, cover her landscape, and then run and laugh back to our house to hide. I was an accessory to the crime. I not only hid my son, but I also harbored his friends. Yard rolling was messy harmless fun. Sometimes they got caught and had to clean it all up. Unfortunately, the kid who lived in the rolled house usually had to clean it up. Our kids only rolled the houses of friends. It wasn't meanness; it was amusement.

When my girls were in high school, there was a football game between two rival high schools in town, and after the game we turned the corner on the street where we lived and spotted our yard under a blizzard of white tissue. The culprits had used over 100 rolls of toilet paper and thrown thousands of cotton swabs all over the yard. The worse part? It rained. Fortunately, we identified the comical criminals, and they came the next day to clean it all up.

Matthew's high school had an annual tradition; seniors pulled a big prank the last week of school. Each year the graduating class tried to outdo the senior classes before it. Matthew's senior group decided to collect thousands of plastic balls from fast food restaurants' playground ball crawls. They piled them all in the "pit" at school. The pit is a low area in one of the hallways, and the unspoken rule was that only seniors and their girlfriends/boyfriends could hang out there. That prank trumped the previous year's. Matthew was right in the middle of the action. After their triumphant joke, the seniors returned all of the balls and even bought new ones for some of the restaurants.

It's good when your child brings his friends home and they feel comfortable at your house. If you can be that parent, take advantage of it. Kids will trust you. You get to keep an eye on the kids. You can also hear what's going on in the basement rec room through vents in your kitchen floor! I liked seeing who my children's buddies were. I've always told them, "You become who you hang out with, so choose your friends carefully."

Matthew was full of life. Back then cell phones didn't exist, so he and his buddies all had pagers. They created and memorized elaborate codes to transfer messages to each other. Matthew's friends were athletes, good students, and

Christians who attended Bible studies. We never worried about what path Matthew would choose when faced with good versus bad decisions. Throughout high school, Matthew dated a girl named Jamie. She was adorable. He had great friends, regularly attended church, and eased through academics. If moral friends, a sweet girlfriend, and good grades weren't insurance enough, there was Young Life. Young Life is a non-denominational Christian organization that works with students to help them follow Jesus Christ and form good values that will help them through life. Matthew was very active in Young Life. We were confident in how we were raising him and assumed that he would never give us any serious trouble. He was the model kid for someone his age.

My husband was a physician, we had a kind son and two sweet, funny daughters, and we lived in a nice house in a safe neighborhood. We were the perfect family.

Shock And Promise

ONE NIGHT, Jim and I were sitting at home watching TV when Matthew and his good friend Brandon walked into our living room. They sat there for a couple of minutes before Brandon looked at Matthew and said, "If you don't tell them, I am going to."

Matthew said, "I smoked some marijuana."

Jim and I were incredibly upset, but we let Matthew do most of the talking. I cried. Then I was suddenly paralyzed with fear. I tried to understand and rationalize the situation. Matthew and his closest friends were in a Bible study and were together a lot. They all went to Frontier Christian camps together. I figured Matthew had some acquaintances outside that group, but I never saw them at our house, and I figured they just socialized at school. I'm assuming that is where he got the pot, but I could be wrong.

I asked him, "Why?"

He answered, "I just wanted to try it."

Matthew apologized over and over. I was certain he was remorseful. He promised to never do it again, and I believed him. Life carried on.

Two years later I found a letter that Matthew's Young Life leader had written to him while Matthew was in high school. In the letter the leader expressed concern for Matthew. He never mentioned suspicion that Matthew was smoking pot, but he alluded to it by writing that Matthew reminded him of himself when he was Matthew's age. He explained that at Matthew's age he questioned everything and took nothing at face value, not even Scripture. Matthew must have been struggling and asking a lot of questions. The Young Life leader wrote that he would continue to pray for Matthew, and that he hoped Matthew would stay on the right path. Matthew had continued to smoke pot, but we didn't know it. I never smelled it, never suspected it, and, of course, never doubted his living room promise.

High School Ends

AFTER GRADUATION, Matthew told Jim and me that he wanted to postpone college and become a Young Life counselor. We immediately said, "No," and sent Matthew just across town to The University of Tennessee in Knoxville. In retrospect, I guess that wasn't a good decision. Perhaps he was trying to choose the right path. Perhaps wanting to be a Young Life counselor was his youthful attempt to hold himself accountable. After one semester Matthew had two A's and one F. His English teacher failed him, accusing him of plagiarism. Matthew swore he wrote the paper. I can't imagine Matthew cheating because he always earned high marks in English. He had no *need* to cheat. English teachers traditionally complimented his work. Matthew dropped most of his classes. His only good grades were in one-hour credits: racquetball and bowling. Jim refused to pay for the next semester. He thought Matthew simply hadn't tried and said he wasn't paying for "nonsense." We suspected too much partying was going on but did not think marijuana was an issue. Jim said, "I'll pay as long as you try. If you stop trying, I'll stop paying." He suggested Matthew take a break, earn money, and pay his own way if he decided to go back. Jim also committed that, if Matthew did well, we would pay tuition again.

He told everyone he wanted to go back to school. I thought all was right with the world. He had a great girl and was headed in the right direction. Matthew did return to campus the following semester, but his schoolwork tanked. We couldn't figure out what was wrong. Matthew had never goofed off in school. The only consistency in his life was his relationship with Jamie.

Working For Mom

AT THE TIME, I MANAGED an apartment complex. Matthew asked if he could work there. Matthew also talked me into hiring one of his friends. Their work included painting, performing simple repairs, landscaping, and completing paperwork for me. Matthew worked eight to five, but his hours sometimes varied as I was pretty lax as long as he got all the work done. If he did projects on nights or weekends, he earned comp time during the week. Matthew was a quick learner. I figured he didn't want to do building maintenance for a living long-term, and I hoped the experience would help him take college more seriously. But something wasn't quite right.

Each morning Matthew came into my office to get his orders for the day. Often, I was on the phone and he had to wait. Countless times, I watched him nod off while I finished phone calls. I asked him if he had stayed out too late. He told me what I wanted to hear, "I'm just tired, Mom."

Increasingly, he nodded off, sometimes even *while* I was talking to him. Hoping to get him to bed earlier, I gave Matthew more outside work and manual labor to keep him busy. Soon, he began not answering his cell phone when I called. Any time I expressed concern that I couldn't reach him, Matthew said what I wanted to hear, "Sorry, Mom. I left it in the car." I found out later that he wasn't telling the truth.

Theft

I WAS PAYING bills one night in my home office when I opened up a notice from the bank. I was overdrawn $2,000 and checks were bouncing! I couldn't believe it. I was instantly furious with the bank and worried that more checks would be returned and that my credit would be ruined. I immediately called the bank. I'm ashamed to say I was impolite toward the lady who answered. I demanded that the bank make everything good and write all of the companies to whom they had returned checks. Then she informed me that several of the checks had been written out of numerical sequence. I asked, "Who are the checks written to?"

She said, "Matthew Seals." All of the checks had been handwritten to him, supposedly signed by me, in the amount of either $100, $200, or $300. They added up to $2,000. I told her I was sorry and that I would check into it. I got off the phone and called Matthew. He was at the movie theater and went out into the hallway to call me back. I guess he had been waiting on that phone call. He said he would take Jamie home and come straight there. I can't explain how upset I was. Before he got there, I tried my best to figure out why he wrote those checks. I wondered if he had gotten into gambling or if he had charged up a bunch of credit cards and was behind on payments. It never occurred to me that he was using drugs. Never.

When Matthew got to my house, I was still sitting at my desk in my office. He walked up to my desk and said, "I have a problem."

I naively scolded him as any mother might, "You sure do!"

He said, "No, Mom, I've got a drug problem."

I remember it like it was yesterday, but I can't adequately articulate the impact his statement had on me. Stunned. Mad. Confused. Heartbroken. Terrified. Matthew explained that he started drinking alcohol and smoking marijuana during his senior year of high school. Then, a "friend" introduced him to OxyContin, and shortly after that, things got out of his control. When he was standing before me at my office desk, I didn't believe what he was telling me. It couldn't be true. He had been hiding his problem in plain sight. He was a functioning addict. A stranger was standing in front of me, a stranger who possessed my son's body. A stranger who promised his parents he wouldn't touch drugs again. A stranger who stole from our family. I had no idea who I was dealing with.

Matthew was deeper into addiction than anyone knew. He was spiraling out of control, alone, submerged in substance and secrecy.

When Matthew admitted his problem to me, I asked if Jamie knew. He said she didn't. I told him either he had to tell her or I would. Telling Jamie scared him much more than telling me. They had been dating for years, and she didn't have a clue about his problem. Jamie had been studying abroad for a while, so she missed the clues.

Naturally, Matthew feared Jamie would leave him. She was an ethical, convicted girl, and he didn't think she would understand or tolerate such a horrific habit. I, too, figured she would run as soon as Matthew told her, but when Matthew confessed his addiction, Jamie didn't run.

Detoxing At Home

AFTER MATTHEW CONFESSED his opiate addiction, I asked him, in my complete naiveté, "Can you quit on your own or should you go to a rehabilitation center?" I had no idea how addicts become clean. He said if he could go through withdrawals he would be fine. We decided he should detox at home. We told the girls that Matthew had the flu, thinking we were keeping them from knowing the ugly truth.

Matthew stayed in our bonus room for several days. It was awful. It was like suffering from the flu one thousand times over. He endured stomach cramps, fevers, profuse sweating, diarrhea, constipation, shivers, and vomiting to the point of throwing up bile. His pain was horrendous. He was deathly sick for five days. I thought we were safe once that nightmare ended. Again, in my naiveté, I thought, *Who in the world would go through that and then go back to drugs?* Relieved and believing Matthew was finally clean, I looked forward to his future and his life being good again. Once you are clean and drugs are out of your system, it is over, right?

Thanksgiving

THANKSGIVING WAS A WEEK LATER. We always have a happy, typical, traditional Thanksgiving dinner. I look forward to Thanksgiving, planning what to cook, and making sure I fix a favorite dish for everyone. I took great care every year to create lasting memories because I knew that when my children got older, it would be harder and harder to bring them together at the same time. I felt so blessed that year. I was "thankful" for my prayers and my good fortune. Little did I know that by the end of the night I would again be worried about Matthew.

Around that colorful, food-filled table, we looked like a Norman Rockwell painting. Each family member stated what he or she was thankful for, then I said grace. If I had it to do over again, we would have made religious practices, like saying grace, more routine in our home. We attended church but didn't pray over meals at the table except at Thanksgiving, Christmas, and Easter. During the meal we drew names for Christmas presents. After the meal we played games and had fun being together. That year, the sweet traditions went off without a hitch. Thanksgiving was happy and normal. We were all together, Matthew was "clean," his girlfriend was content, the girls were laughing, my husband and Matthew enjoyed each other, and all was well in the world.

Later in the evening, Matthew and Jamie left, Courtney and Kimberly went upstairs to their rooms, Jim relaxed to watch college football, and, of course, I cleaned up the kitchen. Earlier in the day, I'd left a $20 bill on the counter by the back door. As I tidied the area, I noticed that the $20 was missing. I remembered setting it there but couldn't figure out what happened to it. I asked Jim if he picked it up. He didn't. I asked both girls if they saw it or picked it up and they said they didn't. I called Matthew on the phone, and he said he didn't see it or get it, either. I then doubted myself, but I just *knew* it had been there that morning. I rationalized, *Maybe Matthew needed the money but was afraid to ask for it because he didn't want me to think he was taking it to buy drugs. Yes, he is just short on cash. He went through absolute hell LAST week. There is no way he plans to go back to using. That is completely illogical. Whoever took it must really need it. Maybe I never set it there.* My heart said one thing but my mind told me he had lied. So why lie? If he just needed some money and had asked, I would have given it to him. But his lying about it was a bad sign. I didn't want to face the truth.

Like so many addicts, my son had relapsed only a week after he detoxed. I didn't see much of Matthew for the next month, except for Christmas.

My office was in one of our apartment buildings at the time. I allowed Matthew to move into the apartment across from my office. One day I saw two guys knocking on Matthew's door. I had never seen these guys before. I knew Matthew wasn't home, so I opened my office door and asked the two young guys what they wanted. They told me they were looking for the guy who lived in that apartment. I told them he wasn't there. They left, but a few minutes later I saw them walking behind the building and sneaking around the backside of Matthew's apartment. I went outside and confronted them again. I asked them to leave or I would have to call the police. Wanting to make sure they left, I walked to the front of the building where they'd first entered. I spotted them looking inside Matthew's car. One of them held a tire tool. Annoyed, I asked them what in the world they were doing. One of the guys hatefully answered me.

He said that Matthew owed him some money and he was there to collect, no matter how he had to do it. He said he was looking for something of value in Matthew's car or he was going to take the tire tool and destroy the whole vehicle. At that moment, I realized they were drug dealers. I asked them how much Matthew owed them. They said $80. (Talk about honor among thieves. Those guys could have claimed Matthew owed $1,000, and it would not have surprised me.) I bargained with them and told them I would pay his debt if they promised to never come back. They agreed. I gave them $80 and they left.

At one point, Matthew went to live with two guys he went to school with. One of those friends called me on the phone and told me Matthew stole $200 from him. Matthew wrote a check on the friend's bank account. The friend planned to press charges because that was the only way the bank could get his money back for him. I begged him not to. He said he would not press charges as long as he got his money back. I gave him the money. He dropped the charges.

I know Jamie must have loved my son very much to stay by him while he was abusing drugs. She opened her home, her parents' home, to Matthew and let him live there for a while. Matthew moved out when he felt he couldn't/shouldn't stay there any longer because addiction was consuming him. After that, I was never sure where he was sleeping. I suspected he was either staying with other drug abusers or living in his car. I didn't know then that Matthew often put his thoughts on paper. I eventually found several of his writings. This is one.

Everyone has his or her own personal struggles. Some of us are at war with an addiction of one form or another. Some are fighting gambling addictions, others fight addictions to sex, shopping, food, alcohol and drugs.

I have been battling an addiction to drugs for some time now and must admit that it is a war in which I am losing.

I wish that I could write about how well my recovery is going and how wonderful it is to finally be sober. This could not be further from the truth. Instead, I can only write about the struggles I am going through and my emotions as I go through them.

Addiction Doesn't Discriminate

I GET UPSET WHEN PEOPLE say addiction is a choice. Yes, an addict does "choose" to take that first pill or snort or hit, but no one "chooses" to become an addict. No one *wants* to be chained, broken, and incarcerated by dependence on a substance. Who *wants* to be an outcast from society? Who *wants* to lose his family? Who *wants* to be an addict?

I could not figure out how to help Matthew, so I tried to figure out addiction. I began researching everything about substance abuse, and I came to many conclusions. I learned that detoxing is only one of many steps to recovery. I also learned that detoxing at home is not only dangerous, but it is also ineffective.

The world attaches unfair negativity to the word itself: *addict*. An addict is someone who is addicted to a substance. By that definition, there are countless addictions in our world today, but none of the users are considered addicts. If you are addicted to nicotine, you are a smoker. If you are addicted to alcohol, you are an alcoholic. If you are addicted to food, you are an overeater. Maybe that's because those substances are legal. Smokers, alcoholics, and overeaters can feed their addictions in broad daylight wherever they are. There should be a new name attached to drug addicts. A name that gives them consideration and hope.

Again, I am not a physician or a therapist, but one should never underestimate the power of a distressed and determined mother. My guess is that there are reasons some people become addicts and some don't. Is it a genetic predisposition? I've read that the genes people are born with account for about half of their chance of addiction. Addiction is a neurological disease that blocks the addict from thinking logically when he is craving drugs or alcohol. Dopamine plays a big role. When a person uses drugs, the dopamine in the brain increases. An addict has lower levels of dopamine than normal. An addict needs more of a certain drug to lessen pain; whereas, a person with normal levels of dopamine does not need as much. The addict's brain craves more of whatever increased the dopamine. When this is passed down genetically, from one family member to the next, relatives must be extra careful when using prescribed medications and when drinking alcohol. Just like any other disease that might run in your family, you have to take care of yourself and realize you are at risk.

When people have genetic predispositions to heart disease or diabetes, people sympathize with them. Whether they eat healthy, exercise, and use caution or do none of the above, people sympathize with them. They don't criticize them, shame them, and family and friends do not shun them. They feel badly for them. My father was an alcoholic, but people didn't understand what I went through living with him. His addiction was accepted as unfortunate, but not unusual. My father didn't have to steal to get drunk every day. Alcohol is cheap. He had to drink more and more to get drunk. Alcoholism is a disease, and people accept it as a disease.

Addiction to illegal drugs like heroin, cocaine, and meth is not acceptable because it's a dirty disease. Let me tell you that living with an alcoholic and watching him hit my mother was no pretty picture. It was extremely dirty and extremely hurtful to a young child. I have mental scars that will never go away. Matthew's ordeal ripped those scars wide open.

The Army

MATTHEW TRIED TO STAY AWAY from drugs, but the pull was so intense he knew he needed to try something drastic. In January, I was out of town and Matthew called to find out where his birth certificate was. I asked him why in the world he needed it, and he told me he had joined the United States Armed Forces. He felt that if he got away from Knoxville, he could stay clean. I've read that it's not uncommon for guys to join the military to stay clean.

He did great during basic training. Matthew wasn't using drugs during that time. I'm pretty sure it would have been impossible for anyone to go through that rigorous training and use drugs. Our family drove to Fort Benning in Columbus, Georgia, to see him graduate. We were so proud of him. Not only did we (Jim, Courtney, Kimberly and I) go, but also Jamie and several of his best friends from high school went. They had all watched him struggle. I was so appreciative that Matthew's friends drove eight hours to see him graduate. We were all so proud of him and what he had accomplished.

Matthew wrote letters at night in the dark when lights were out in the barracks because he didn't have time during the day to write. I suppose that was the only time he had to reflect. He was probably homesick. He wrote to his sisters and me, and I'm sure he wrote to Jamie, too. In his letters to Courtney and Kimberly, he encouraged them to make better decisions than he had.

Matthew was raised in church, was intelligent, and he had the tools to work hard and succeed at anything. The Army was good for him for a little while. Perhaps he was afraid he might go into combat, or perhaps the Holy Spirit was working in him. I don't know, but Matthew was baptized while enlisted. I was elated when he told me. My children were raised Presbyterian and then Methodist, both of which allow for babies to be christened or for believers to be baptized at a later time. I was raised Baptist, so I never really thought about "christening" my children. I figured when they came of age to choose, they would do so. Being baptized is not a requirement to get into heaven, as salvation is a gift that is received by grace through faith. Baptism is an outward act of testimony to others as a result of your salvation. If you want to be saved, all you have to do is accept Jesus into your heart.

Even though Matthew strayed from his teachings, he came back to them. I congratulated myself and thought of Proverbs 22:6 (ESV): "Train up a child in the way he should go; even when he is old he will not depart from it."

AWOL

MATTHEW LEFT FORT BENNING and went to Fort Gordon to do his Advanced Individual Training. It was then when he met some guys in his unit who introduced him to heroin. Once he started using heroin, he was on his way to almost irreversible self-destruction.

Matthew would sometimes drive home on a Friday evening and go back on Sunday evening. A couple of times, he brought his army buddies home—I now know they were the ones who introduced him to heroin. They would go out at night and come in very late. They slept in our basement. I kidded myself, thinking they were just out having a good time and he was showing them Knoxville.

One reason Matthew started coming home was because he missed Jamie and wanted to see her, but he also came home to contact his old drug connections. Out of nowhere he came home one weekend and announced that he wasn't going back to the army. Then he drove off. I called his cell phone and I begged and pleaded with him to go back to base.

After many minutes, he assured me he was on the interstate and he was going to go back. He lied. I have no idea where he ended up, but it wasn't back at the base.

Being the "good" codependent mother, I emailed his sergeant, and asked him how long Matthew could stay home before he was considered AWOL (absent without official leave) and how much trouble he was in. His sergeant was extremely nice and promised that if Matthew returned within 24 hours, he wouldn't punish him. Matthew didn't go straight back. He stayed out for two weeks and attempted to detox again on his own.

Jim was repulsed the entire time Matthew went through withdrawals in our home the first time. I was worried about how he would react to the awful news about Matthew's relapse. It turned out that I had every right to be concerned. Jim lost it. Several days later Matthew was in the basement in our home and detoxing for the second time. Jim went downstairs and confronted Matthew. In front of Jamie and me, Jim said, "I am disgusted. I want you to leave. As long as you are doing drugs, leave our home and do NOT come back here."

Hysterical, I followed Matthew and Jamie as they walked outside. He looked at me through his car window and said, "I will never be back."

It must be difficult for people to understand this, but Jim and I didn't discuss Matthew's addiction. Jim thought drug addicts were nasty and distasteful. I didn't want to hear criticism of my child, especially when I was so worried. I didn't even tell my mother what was happening. To this day, she still knows nothing about Matthew's addiction. She would have been heartbroken, and I could not put her through that pain and have to console her all the time. I already had enough emotions to deal with.

Matthew actually returned to his Army base. When confronted by a commanding officer, Matthew admitted he had a drug problem, but supervisors didn't believe him. Matthew was hoping to get help. The officer told Matthew he could go to a clinic once a week and speak with someone—as if a weekly conversation with anyone could solve the problem. Matthew needed much more. The military officers soon recognized that, and I guess they did not want to deal with drugs or anyone using. They released Matthew without any ramifications, and he came back to Knoxville. I think the Army today is much better equipped to handle drug issues.

Out Of Bounds

I KNEW MATTHEW was back in Knoxville, but I didn't know where. Desperate to see him and make sure he was alive, I drove dangerous streets in the middle of the night looking for his car, praying I would see it just so I'd know he was still alive. My car was expensive. I figured some people might see it and think it held a drug dealer. I knew that there were turf wars and that someone could shoot at my car. I also figured the car would be a good theft target, which also put me in danger, but I didn't care. I wondered where he bought drugs, what kind of people he was with, how they did drugs, and where they did them. I not only worried about him overdosing but also about being arrested, beaten up, robbed, or killed. I could only imagine the worst-case scenarios even though I didn't want to visualize them. It's probably better that I never got answers to those questions.

In all my wee-hour searches, I never found Matthew's car. Maybe that was a blessing because I was so scared and upset, I might have stayed in front of a drug dealer's house and waited on Matthew to come out. Maybe I would have gone inside. He would have been extremely angry. My being there would have been dangerous for him, too. Dealers wouldn't want me to know where drugs were being sold. They might beat Matthew senseless to send me a warning and keep me from telling police about them. I drove around like that only when I hadn't heard from him in a while. I wanted to see my son's car somewhere, anywhere. If I did, then I knew he was alive. I was scared in those neighborhoods, but not nearly as scared as I was of my son being dead. Jamie asked to go with me one night so I wasn't driving around alone. She came over and we went out around 2:00 a.m. searching for his car. I found out fourteen years later that Jamie was also driving around on nights by herself looking for him.

When you love an addict, your desperation to lay eyes on him or her is overwhelming. So is the anger when you do—anger that your loved one "chooses" to stay in addiction rather than try to take help and get clean. I felt like my journey with Matthew was a "heartship" not a hardship. My heart was breaking, and I didn't know what it was going to take to put the pieces back together again.

I kept my phone with me at all times. Part of me was afraid it would ring, and another part of me was afraid it wouldn't. I didn't know which was worse. The phone was my worst enemy and my best friend. There were days when I wouldn't hear anything from him, not even a text. I would message Jamie to see if she had heard from him. I would type, "Son, please just let me know you are okay. I love you." Most of the time I got nothing back but when he did respond, I thanked God. If he didn't respond, fear overwhelmed me. My heart almost leapt out of my chest when he replied with a simple, "I'm okay."

I wanted desperately to tell him face to face that I loved him. Matthew had a favorite T-shirt with the logo for the rock band Rage Against the Machine. I found the shirt in his room and wore it every night. For some strange reason, it made me feel closer to him, like I could protect him if I had on his favorite shirt. It was part of my armor. Matthew was desperate, too. About that time, he wrote the following:

Addiction is such a difficult thing to understand because it defies all rational thinking.

Who would willingly take part in self-destructive behavior on a daily basis?

What kind of person chooses to live in a self-loathing prison of misery?

Who would let go of everything they have worked so hard to earn and every gift they have been given to hold on to nothing?

What kind of person would lie to, steal from, ignore, abandon, and hurt those who love him only to embrace another person who would do the same horrible things to him without remorse?

What type of living, breathing, human being would choose captivity over freedoms, pain over pleasure, loneliness over companionship, enemies over family and friends, struggle over peace, a temporary high over a lasting sense of relief, and dying over living?

I will tell you what type of person—a drug addict.

I know these things are true, because I have chosen those things myself. And I am in fact, a drug addict. I have asked myself these very same questions. And, although I know what the answers are, I do not know why.

Empty

AT ONE POINT MATTHEW CALLED me to see if I had an empty apartment he could use for a few nights. We did, so I told him I would unlock the door. It was painful for me to do that because the apartment was completely bare. I knew he would sleep on the floor. During one of Matthew's lowest points, he wrote these thoughts:

In my search for answers concerning my addiction, I tend to end up back in the familiar arms of anger, self-loathing, and self-pity. I try my best not to sit around feeling sorry for myself, but sometimes I cannot help but feel that I have been dealt an unfair hand in the poker game of life. What I need to realize is, even if that is the case, I still need strength enough to throw in my chips and courage enough to play my hand. However, if poker chips represent my strength and playing my hand is symbolic of my courageousness, at the present time I am dead broke and about to fold.

Perhaps I have spent too much time asking God to deal me a better hand and not enough time asking him to help me deal with the hand I already have.

Again, he left the apartments . . . probably because he didn't want me checking up on him. He was in a really bad place. I didn't know where he was staying half the time and really didn't want to know.

Eventually, he moved in with two of his friends who lived in the apartment above my office. But, I had no idea he was up there. One day I went up the stairs to check on a vacant apartment that happened to be across the hall from Matthew's friends' unit. As I put the key in the door, Matthew came out of the friends' apartment. We made eye contact, but he stared a hole right through me. He did not speak one word. His eyes locked on mine and stayed locked as he walked down the flight of stairs then out of sight.

I didn't recognize that person.

My fun-loving, always smiling, thoughtful son was gone. I saw empty eyes. Darkness. A darkness I had never seen before and never want to see again. I was terrified. Matthew's soul was missing. I met evil face to face. I met The Beast.

I opened the door to the empty apartment I was going in to check on and dropped straight to my knees. I told God I had looked into the eyes of Satan and prayed that He would remove the Beast that was inside Matthew. I told God that I was terrified.

Did my son feel abandoned by me? By our family? I prayed that he would know he was never abandoned. My thoughts were with him every moment of every single day. I loved him with all my heart.

Modern-Day Demonic Possession

I NEVER HATED MATTHEW when he was using. I hated The Beast, the lying, the stealing, the pain, the hopelessness and the powerlessness Matthew must have felt. I loved him so much but hated his ways. I missed him a lot. I have never lost a child to death, but I am sure addiction is as close as it gets. To me, he was dying little by little every day, and I couldn't see him or be his mother. I was in perpetual mourning with no relief in sight.

The reasoning part of the brain is not fully developed until around age 25. Before the age of 25, a lot of bad decisions can be made; however, those decisions do not have to define a person for the rest of his life. The decision to take drugs in the first place is a choice, but the drug changes the structure of the brain, which over time, can affect choices to make the right decisions. It has nothing to do with willpower, strength of character, morality, or intelligence. Many people believe if a person wants to quit abusing drugs, he should just be able to do it. If that were the case, there would be no addicts.

"The Beast" is the name I gave to Matthew's addiction because it possessed him like a demon. It took everything from him. It took control of his mind, his body, his thoughts, his feelings, his emotions, and his soul. I didn't recognize my son. Matthew appeared perpetually angry. I was angry, too. I was angry that The Beast wouldn't let Matthew go, that it had more of a hold on him than I did. I was angry at God for not helping me help Matthew get well. I would have paid any ransom in the world to bring my child back.

You know The Beast when you see it. It is in control. If you let it get close, it will control you, too. The Beast has no empathy, just like the pain it causes. It lies, steals and manipulates. The Beast is dark and powerful. Matthew wrote:

I am lost
And cannot find my way home
I do believe that I AM loved
But don't know how to BE loved
I wonder what other people think about me
Do they think I will get better?
Do I?
Have they given up on me?
Have I?
Do they care?
Do I?

The Beast Means Business

I THOUGHT I WAS HELPING my son in all of the things I did. Fearing he would doubt my love, I caved when he came to me for anything. I thought I was keeping him alive. I thought that eventually he would change back to the old Matthew. As a mother, I trusted that my efforts and love were strong enough and that I was taking the right action. My motives were pure. I could not understand why "I" could not get him to stop. Didn't he realize how much I cared? How much I cried? How much I hurt? How much I worried? How much sleep I lost? How much I needed him to stop? Of course he did. It was one of the reasons he didn't want to see me or talk to me. He felt guilty, but he also felt out of control. The Beast had a stronger hold on him than I did. The Beast wouldn't allow Matthew to listen to anyone. It made Matthew feel better for only short spurts of time with toxic highs. Then, when Matthew tried to stop, he became physically ill and The Beast convinced him it could help him feel better again. Most people can't imagine a substance having that much control over their lives. Jim and I couldn't. Before addiction, Matthew had a sound grip on emotions and choices. He took nothing at face value. He was logical, reasonable, and liked facts. If The Beast could take control of Matthew, I knew it would be hard to defeat. It wreaked havoc in Matthew's life by steering his every thought and movement. In my heart, I knew I couldn't fight the enemy alone, and I knew a stronger power than The Beast existed. The Beast wanted Matthew to think all hope was gone, but I knew better. No matter what mistakes Matthew made, no matter what The Beast knew about Matthew's weaknesses, Matthew did not have to live in the dark. In my frustration and loneliness, I penned a poem about The Beast.

The Beast

Have you ever been in such
A deep, dark place that you
Didn't see a way out?
No light? No hope?
Total darkness is where The Beast lives.
He doesn't want to let you go.
He will take your will and then your soul.
The Best would love to keep you there—fear him.

But know and trust God
To bring in the light because
God is the way out.
He has always been there
And He will never let you go.
He will protect you, give you hope,
Heal you, and show you a way out.
God would love to take you there—trust Him.

Enabling

MY LOVE FOR MATTHEW WAS ENDLESS, but my love wasn't enough to conquer The Beast. Actually, I *assisted* The Beast in Matthew's self-destruction by enabling my son. I did so by lying for Matthew when he worked for me. He was often late, and I knew the drugs caused him to oversleep. When he lied or didn't communicate with our family, I made excuses as to why he didn't call or come over. Matthew asked me for money to pay his bills because he was "short and his utilities might be cut off." He didn't have money for gas, he didn't have money for food, he didn't have money to pay his car note, he didn't have money to pay his phone bill, etc. I gave him money for all of the above, time after time.

I *let* him steal. If he took something from the house, I lied or didn't tell Jim. He pawned things out of his own apartment that I had bought for him. I went to the pawn stores and bought everything back. Usually, I gave the stuff back to Matthew. He would turn around and pawn it again as soon as he needed money. I bought and re-bought things several times. What the heck was I thinking?

I have always been accessible to my children, and I always will be. Parents are made that way. We feed and rock babies at all hours of the day and night. We lose sleep because nothing is more important. We play games that we may not necessarily want to play but we do it to make them happy. We are room mothers. We attend all school functions. We help with homework. We go to every sporting event and cheer them on. We are sometimes "that mother" who yells louder than every other mother. We hold back tears of pride when there is a special accomplishment. We are the Tooth Fairy, the Easter Bunny, and Santa Claus. We wholeheartedly, immediately, without reservation, commit to loving and protecting our children from pregnancy onward. I have learned that there are distinct, crucial differences between helping and enabling. Enabling someone makes it easier for him to continue making bad choices, exhibiting destructive behavior, and floundering in addiction. If Courtney told me she was planning to rob a bank, would I volunteer to drive the getaway car? Of course not, so why did I fund Matthew's drug problem? Parents enable, thinking we are helping. We fear that if we don't help our children how they want, we'll lose the relationship entirely.

Enabling drains you not only financially, but also emotionally and physically. If you love someone who is out of control and you find yourself taking responsibility for the person's actions, you are an enabler and you lose control, too. The worst part is that the enabler is usually more affected and more upset than the one being enabled. You worry. You spend. You lose sleep. You hurt others. You obsess over consequences. You are held hostage by the whole situation, especially when the person you are enabling makes you feel guilty if you don't help (enable) him.

You enable out of fear and from a place of love but enabling makes you part of the problem. Even though you are "helping" from a place of genuine, well-intentioned love, you are not moving your child toward a cure. You are making the disease worse, and your misguided love turns into all-consuming fear.

Second-Hand Shame

WHEN YOUR CHILD IS ADDICTED to drugs, you don't go around telling your friends. I felt shame, embarrassment, and guilt. Guilt is something mothers do very well. We have guilt down to a science. I wondered what I had done, what I could have done differently, or what I shouldn't have done at all. I was sure Matthew's addiction was somehow my fault. Thus, *I* had to fix it. There are those words again: *I fix it.* I thought, *I'm his mother. That's my job. Mothers make things right for their children.* I was afraid if I didn't do something to "fix Matthew," something would happen to him, and I would mourn with guilt for the rest of my life.

Because of the stigma often associated with drug abuse, I felt like I couldn't talk to anyone because no one could understand and everyone might judge me as a mother and Matthew as a person. During my rampant research, I read an article in *Psychology Today*. Addiction expert Carolyn Ross, MD, M.P.H wrote that 50 percent of Americans have a friend or family member with an opiate addiction. The majority of heroin users started with prescription pain pills. At the time Ross conducted the research, approximately 90 Americans died every day as a result of an opiate overdose, most commonly from heroin. According to the CDC, the figure for overdoses in 2017 was approximately 200 a day. According to Barry Meier, author of the book *Pain Killer,* in 2016, 64,000 Americans died from drug overdoses. OxyContin first appeared in the mid-1990's and was considered the new "wonder" drug for pain. OxyContin was not a "wonder" drug. It was the gateway drug to the most devastating public-health disaster of the 21st century. According to a *Vox* article written in 2017, more Americans died of drug overdoses in 2016 than died in the entirety of the Vietnam War. And, according to *Times,* 2017 was worse than in 2016. In 2017, the number exceeded 70,000. I recently read that the national average life expectancy is dropping due to young people dying of drug overdose. Also, according to a report dated April 14, 2019, from the National Safety Council, Americans' odds of dying from an accidental opioid overdose are higher than the odds of dying from a motor vehicle crash.

With those statistics it stands to reason that I could reach out to talk to *anyone* because probably more than half of my friends knew someone struggling in addiction. Millions of Americans abuse or are dependent on drugs and alcohol, but unfortunately, just like an addict, I felt completely alone.

Can you imagine what it must feel like to believe you can't stop? Can you imagine feeling like you are going to lose your job, your family, your friends, your home, your children?

I tried to put on a brave front in the midst of my adversity. I didn't want people to know the pain my family was suffering. I went through life day-to-day carrying the burden by myself.

While Matthew was helplessly immersed in addiction, I continued to go through the motions of life. I drove home every day after work. I smiled and waved to neighbors. As I made these routine, polite, seemingly happy gestures, I thought of the irony in my life. To others, I guess I have appeared put together and content. No one ever asked me if anything was wrong. I fulfilled obligations and acted as normally as I could when I wasn't alone. In reality, I was falling apart. I wrote a poem to capture such irony.

I Am Just One Mother

I am just one mother
But I know I am not alone.
I am your friend and your neighbor.
I wave and smile as I
Pass by you because it is
The neighborly thing to do.
I don't know your pain and
You don't know mine.
I will tell you how wonderful
My family is and I will listen
To you talk about yours.
I don't know if your story is full of
Lies like mine is,
But who am I to judge?

I wonder if I am a good friend
Because there are days
That I certainly don't feel like
I am a good mother.
The Beast has taken my
Son and he is trying to
Take me as well.
Do you know the Beast?
He will try to move into your
Neighborhood and will want to
Be your friend.
You are just one mother
But you are not alone.

We are not meant to go through life alone or struggle alone. When we isolate ourselves and don't let God in, we are making it easy for Satan, or as I called Matthew's addiction—The Beast—to step in and fill that void. He loves it when we isolate ourselves. You can't hide your suffering from God. He already knows our sufferings. He is patient. He waits.

Loving Him To Death

AS MATTHEW SANK DEEPER AND DEEPER into drugs, I sank deeper and deeper into guilt. I told him I loved him every moment that he crossed my mind. I called and texted him. My heart exploded anytime he sent back a message telling me he loved me, too.

Those messages were few. Matthew seldom responded, which I attributed to his own overpowering guilt. I know he hated being entombed by heroin. He hated that he was causing his family and friends such anguish. He understood, academically, that he was taking insane risks, but his emotional state and chemical dependence were a grave duo. According to what I've read and experienced with Matthew, drug addicts don't want to feel guilty or responsible for hurting others. Those feelings of shame and despair only led Matthew to seek more drugs, more highs.

My mental existence was a living, exhausting, lonely hell. I was powerless as I watched my son make life-altering decisions that cost him everything. I was consumed with worry that Matthew would get arrested, overdose, or die. I hated to see the sun go down. Peaceful rest was impossible. I was afraid I would sleep through a text message or a phone call, so I kept my phone volume on maximum and kept the phone pressed between my cheek and my pillow all night long. I slept upstairs in my office on a couch most evenings. If Matthew needed me, I was ready. There were days and weeks when I wouldn't hear anything from him—not even a text. He called Jamie more often than he did me. I think he still wanted to know she was there and not giving up. When I couldn't locate Matthew, I found peace of mind only by convincing myself over and over that he must be with her. I was grateful for her. She was patient. She was kind. She was STRONG. She was his guardian angel.

I constantly thought, *What can I do?* I prayed. I worried. I cried. I called drug rehab centers the few times Matthew was in my office. The centers' representatives all asked me the same question, "Why are you calling? Your son should be making this call." I told them I was just trying to help. They told me that helping him would mean leaving it to Matthew make the call. I didn't really understand what they meant. I didn't care. I was frantic.

During that time, I felt I was being a terrible wife and mother. Exhausted in my secret hell, I gave everything I could to my husband when he was around, and I gave everything I could to my girls when I was with them, but I didn't have much to give. Inside, I was dying. I was lost. I felt like a total failure.

Matthew called me out of the blue one day and said, "Mom, I'm hungry. I haven't eaten in days." I asked him what he wanted and he said Wendy's cheeseburgers. I bought him two cheeseburgers and a Coke. I met him in a parking lot. My heart broke as I watched him inhale the food. Normally, it's a simple joy to feed a hungry boy, but in that moment, I had never felt so sorry for anyone in my life. He said only, "Thank you, Mom." He drove off in one direction. I drove off in the other direction. I was crying so hard that I had to pull off the road so I wouldn't wreck.

I knew that if one or both of us didn't make some changes, my worst fears would surely come true. Yes, I feared for his life. While I knew I could not stop his addiction, I knew that I could stop myself from playing a part. I needed help even if Matthew wasn't willing to get any. One addict can take a whole family down. I finally broke my silence and confided in a friend.

Help From A Friend

AFTER THINGS GOT SO OUT OF CONTROL, I needed someone to talk to. I had never felt so alone. I could have talked more with Jamie, but I knew she was already having to deal with too much herself, and I didn't want to trouble her with my problems, issues, and concerns. My burden was so heavy that I needed help to carry it. I just happened to be with my dear friend Terri one day when I was feeling so low and so alone. It helped to be able to say something out loud and not hold it all in. When I confessed what was going on, Terri was sympathetic and listened without offering advice. She called me a little later and asked if I had ever heard about Celebrate Recovery. I'm not sure how Terri knew about Celebrate Recovery, but I am so thankful that she did.

Once I started sharing my story and my fears, it became easier and easier to talk about Matthew's addiction with her. I maintained my secret, for the most part, because I couldn't tolerate judgment.

One of my biggest reasons for not talking to anyone besides Terri was concern about how people would feel about Matthew. I wondered, *How will they label my child? Will they feel sorry for him? For me? Will they criticize us? Will they shun us? Will people's comments make me feel worse? How can people possibly relate? How can they even help?*

Addiction is a heavy, dark, filthy subject. It's almost like you think if you don't talk about it and you don't tell anyone, it will go away and no one will ever find out.

Have you ever noticed that when mothers get together, they share all of the wonderful things their kids are doing? It's like we can't brag enough or be proud enough. Women should be more open with one another and share our sorrows and stresses without judgement. Instead of being annoyed by an in-law or coworker, we should ask her if she needs help. Through all this I have learned not to judge people because I never know what they are going through. If, through conversation or social media, we create these perfect families with perfect husbands and perfect kids, how can someone who is struggling share her issues and ask for help from other women? In that light, I now make an effort not to brag about my kids and grandkids so that a friend has room to open up. Think about it. How does boasting that your child just passed medical boards or got into college or landed a six-figure job help the person to whom you are speaking? My children may not be shining stars to someone else, but they are shining stars to me. I don't need to tell the world all of the wonderful things they do unless someone who really knows them and is truly interested asks.

Guess what? There is no perfect family. There is no perfect spouse. There are no perfect children. We all have been through something in our lives. We all have bad days, weeks, months, or even years. We all need someone in our lives who will just listen and offer support. I didn't need anyone to solve my problems. I couldn't even figure out how to solve them *myself*. I just wanted and needed someone to love me, comfort me, and pray with me. I wanted and needed someone by my side. Terri reacted just like I had hoped she would—with love, support, and most of all, prayers.

I encourage anyone who has a loved one in an addiction to reach out to your closest friends. Reach out for a support group and read as much as you can about addiction.

I took Terri's advice and sought help through Celebrate Recovery at Cokesbury United Methodist Church in Knoxville, Tennessee. I drove there a couple of times but left because I was scared and self-conscious. It took me a long time to walk through those church doors. I remember thinking that people would assume I was there for my own addiction problem. If you have an addict in your family, you DO have an addiction problem.

Believe it or not, some of my friends still don't know our story. The ones who later learned the story asked me why I didn't confide in them. I explained that I was embarrassed and just couldn't find the words.

Because I was so embarrassed, I wasn't even able to tell one of my oldest and dearest friends, Rita. Rita is one of my prayer warriors. She is the least judgmental person I know. I realize now that I could have trusted her to be discreet, but because of my shame and guilt, I remained silent and suffered needlessly when I could have reached out to her for more support. When I finally did tell Rita, she embraced me in affection, encouragement, and continual prayer.

Celebrate Recovery

MATTHEW WAS NOT AT FAULT for having a disease, but he was responsible for seeking treatment. I knew I was responsible for getting treatment for myself. I had to step out of my comfort zone, step over the hurdles of embarrassment and shame, and do something to help myself. I chose to attend the meetings Celebrate Recovery held at Cokesbury United Methodist Church because I needed to be around people who were going through what I was going through. I needed to hear stories of recovery. I needed to hear that my child could heal. I needed hope.

Matthew's addiction was stealing my happiness and ruining my life because I allowed it. Matthew was responsible for his recovery but he was not responsible for mine. I had to take control of that part of my life. You've heard the expression, "If you are at the end of your rope, tie a knot and hang on." I say, "If you are at the end of your rope, pray!" I was at the end of my rope.

Celebrate Recovery started over 26 years ago at Saddleback Church in California with 43 people in attendance the first night. Celebrate Recovery has helped more than 21,000 at that church alone. It is now in over 35,000 churches worldwide. It may have saved my life. I know it saved my sanity once I found out I was not alone in my suffering. I always thought drug addicts were "lowlifes" or "junkies" who came from bad families and lived on the streets. They were unintelligent, bad people who did criminal acts. I had never met a drug addict and as far as I knew, no members of my social circle had ever dealt with addiction. They all had good kids. Good kids didn't become drug addicts. When I pictured a drug addict, I never pictured my son. Celebrate Recovery opened my eyes.

Celebrate Recovery doesn't really tell you what you should or shouldn't do. When you attend their meetings and listen to others' stories, what you should or shouldn't do becomes obvious through lessons, group meetings, and testimonies from others.

There are other programs that tell you to just walk away, to cut addicts off both financially and emotionally. Tough love sounds workable, but in reality, few parents can stomach that approach. It's like being out in the wilderness and having your foot caught in a bear trap. Your only tool is a saw. You know what you must do to survive, but you dwell in pain trying every other possible way before succumbing to the inevitable.

Celebrate Recovery's approach is based on Biblical principles. The program addresses all kinds of addictions and disorders. Most groups meet weekly and are sponsored by churches. If your city has multiple Celebrate Recoveries sites, they usually meet on different nights. My advice to you would be to visit all of them. You can decide to only go once a week to the one you feel the most comfortable attending, or you can go to more than one. Meetings begin with large groups, then attendees break into small groups based on needs.

The small group I attended was the Family Support Group. The first couple of weeks I went, I cried all the way through the large group meeting and all the way through the small group meetings. I couldn't speak in the small group because I was still too embarrassed. Besides, why did I need to speak? Everyone in there was already telling my story! There would be anywhere from 20 to 25 people at the table and every one of them was living the same nightmare. I wasn't special. I was broken like the rest of them. As time went on, I got better at speaking up. Once you go to a few meetings and hear enough stories, you begin to see the big picture. I did notice that loved ones, whether parents, spouses, siblings, or friends, handled addiction so differently. We all needed help. I remember sitting in one meeting and a mother asked the group, "What if I do the wrong thing and my child kills himself? I would have to live with that guilt." I knew how she felt. I felt guilty. I felt like I was already enabling my son to kill himself. Some of the people in our small group were obvious enablers and some were not. When I first started going, I was looking for answers. I was surprised and disappointed when no one told me what to do. The thing is, there is not a one-size fits all solution. What works for one addict may not work for the other. Celebrate

Recovery doesn't harbor judgment or allow advice between participants. They let you share, but no one tells you what to do. You aren't allowed to cross talk or offer solutions to anyone else's problems. I shared that I had tried yelling, bribing, begging, crying, and enabling—none of which had worked for anyone else in my group. While I was willing to try anything, my attempts were pointless. It boiled down to that old saying about the definition of insanity—doing the same thing over and over and expecting a different result. If your child or loved one is in an addiction, you need to get help for yourself. There are groups you can join. Do it for yourself. No matter how strong you think you are, you can't do this alone.

Through the support of other people at Celebrate Recovery and the leaders there, along with wonderful encouragement from my friends Terri and Rita, I got stronger. I no longer felt alone. I can't imagine how I would have coped during that time without Celebrate Recovery. There are other good programs, but I like Celebrate Recovery because it is Christ-centered. I needed the comfort and reassurance of God. I needed His infinite mercy and grace.

Through Celebrate Recovery, I discovered I didn't cause Matthew to use drugs and I couldn't stop him from using drugs. It wasn't about me. I couldn't fix Matthew. Only God could. I don't know why I thought I could do a better job than God. God waited patiently for me to move out of the way and let Him show Matthew mercy and grace. He is the great healer.

Jamie and I actually convinced Matthew to attend Celebrate Recovery several times, which he did, likely out of guilt and to appease Jamie and me. I knew he was high when he was there, but I hoped he still heard the message that he could get clean and stay clean.

A man named Dr. Gil Smith directed the Celebrate Recovery program at that time. Gil is a recovering addict who has an amazing story to tell. He was a United Methodist pastor. He became addicted to alcohol and drugs, which caused him to lose his pastoral credentials. He was living in a Sunday school classroom at the church when a pastor there decided Cokesbury should offer a substance abuse recovery program. Gil, as he became known to all of us, went to the training program at Saddleback Church in California, the home of Celebrate Recovery. He then became the director at Cokesbury where he counseled and inspired close to 400 people every Thursday night.

Gil later relocated to St. Petersburg, Florida, where he launched a Celebrate Recovery ministry. Gil has since retired. The program at Cokesbury has changed and is no longer part of Celebrate Recovery. It is now Recovery at Cokesbury.

One day I hope Gil will write his story to inspire others. He was so helpful to me and connected with Matthew on a level I couldn't. I don't know how I would have made it through the toughest times in my life without having his mentorship and the support, kinship, and resources of Celebrate Recovery.

Signs

PARENTS DON'T WANT TO BELIEVE their children will ever abuse drugs. Reading about the signs of drug addiction is different than actually living them. It's easy to miss the signs when the user is your own child. Maybe parents notice things but ignore them out of fear. Some excuse behavioral changes as "going through a phase," "just being a teen," "I did the same thing when I was her age," or "so-and-so's child did that, too." Parents must be cautious and curious. I thought I was. Parents should monitor who their children's friends are. Matthew had good friends. If you suspect one of your child's friends may be using drugs, chances are your child is, too.

Way back when Matthew admitted that he had tried pot, I really wanted to believe his promise to never do it again. He lived in a solid Christian environment. Matthew had never done anything to lose my trust. He was never late for curfew, his grades were good, he spoke respectfully to Jim and me, and he was loving toward his family. He wanted to be a good son, but he was an addict, and we missed many clues. I have listed some signs of drug addiction that I became aware of in my experience and my research:

*Sudden weight loss
*Changes in academic performance
*Bloodshot eyes
*Enlarged or small pupils
*Insomnia or the opposite—appears sleepy all of the time
*Lack of motivation
*Absence from work or school
*Behavioral problems at work or school
*Irritability, mood swings
*Changes in personality or attitude
*Avoiding friends and family
*Financial problems, always needs money
*Lying and keeping secrets
*Loss of interest in things the person used to care about
*Household items missing

Heroin is highly addictive and overdoses can be fatal. Heroin users may present additional signs of addiction:

*Small pieces of foil with burn marks
*Spoons with burn marks
*Needles
*Shoelaces, rubber bands, or anything that can be tied around the arms
*Lots of lighters
*Cut up straws

*Stomach or muscle cramps or diarrhea
*Track marks on arms or other body parts

It's a lot harder to detect addiction when your child is no longer living at home. I missed the cues but when I did notice signs, I excused them or justified them.

Liars

DRUG ADDICTS ARE MASTER MANIPULATORS. They are professional liars. There is a saying, "How do you know when addicts are lying? When their lips are moving." Matthew lied about everything. He lied about where he was, what he was doing, where his money was going. He lied about his bills and lied about having money stolen. For a very long time, I bought in to all those lies. I even made excuses for him.

Matthew stole from everyone. He even stole from his younger sisters, and he loves them dearly. Even after he stole from them, Kimberly justified it by saying Matthew must have really needed the money to take it from her bank. I replaced the money and told her Matthew had given it to me to give back to her. You could say I was covering for him again, and maybe I was, but I didn't want her to see all the ugliness of her brother's addiction. I wanted to protect her and Courtney from seeing or knowing about The Beast. I didn't want to tarnish their image of Matthew. Their forgiveness had no boundaries just like drug addicts have no boundaries.

If they have grandparents close by, addicts may visit their grandparents more often and "borrow" money. In all of the years during Matthew's turmoil and after, I listened to all kinds of stories. The ones about how grandchildren took advantage of vulnerable grandparents were the hardest to hear. It's hard enough for parents to say no, but almost impossible for grandparents to reject their beloved grandchildren. I am so glad my mother lives in another town because I would have been furious if Matthew had used her for money. Her living on the opposite side of the state also helped me hide the truth from her.

While Matthew was in his addiction, I was also a liar. I tried to act as if nothing was wrong in my life. I was very active in our county, state, and national medical alliance. I was on several boards and held positions on important committees. At one point, I was the chairman of the national membership committee for the American Medical Association Alliance, an organization for spouses of physicians. The group helps communities lead healthy lifestyles. I was heading the effort to recruit members who could further that cause. Isn't it ironic that my life was falling apart while I was trying to help everyone else keep theirs healthy? I guess it doesn't seem strange to other enablers, because that's what we do. It's hard to live two different lives—especially two that are polar opposite. The funny thing to me now is my end goal was to be president of that organization. I had worked from being county president to state president and served on the national level. I was on my way. The next year, instead of being asked to be a director, which would have meant moving closer to being president, I was asked to be membership chairman again because I had done such a great job. Instead of accepting the role, I resigned. It was probably a God wink because if I had been made a director, I would have continued to lead two lives. My goals had to change. My focus needed to be on my family. I walked away from what I perceived to be an important milestone for me and put that energy toward being a good wife and mother.

Old Bad Habits

SOMETIMES WE THINK WE CAN GET AWAY with doing something wrong if no one sees us. Sooner or later doing wrong will catch up with us. If you or a loved one is facing a battle, God can give you the strength you need to overcome whatever it is you are facing, but you must listen and be willing to step out of your comfort zone. Only after you obey God can you move forward. Matthew 6:24 (NIV) reads, "No one can serve two masters." God cannot work in us or in our loved ones if we put something above Him. Matthew was putting drugs before God. I was putting Matthew and my anxiety before God. Our priorities were poisoning the potential of any recovery for Matthew.

Staying clean borders on impossible. There are thousands of stories of addicts who go to detox or rehab or jail and get clean, and there are just as many stories about relapses. I think one of the hardest things for addicts to do, once they are clean, is avoid the friends they had before they got clean. I have seen it many times. When Matthew went back to the friends he hung out with when he was using, he relapsed. In the family support group at Celebrate Recovery, I heard parents say their kids got out of rehab and as soon as they went back to old friends, they relapsed. It is lonely to avoid old friends, especially those who "get it." Addicts may think it's too hard to make new friends or that the healthy relationships they had before using drugs have permanently ended. Matthew fell into this trap, he detoxed but reverted to the same toxic friends.

Jamie called me one day and told me Matthew was at her parents' house but was leaving soon. She knew how upset I was and that I needed to physically see him. I got in my car and raced to her parents' house. I pulled my car up behind his so he couldn't back out and leave before I spoke to him. I forced him to listen to me. When he came to the back of his trunk to put stuff in his car, I said, "I love you and I am praying for you."

He said, "I don't believe in God anymore. I have prayed and prayed that my addiction will go away, but God has done nothing to take it from me."

I couldn't believe what I was hearing from my son, until I realized The Beast was speaking for him. I said, "Matthew, please don't say that. Continue to pray. I will. I love you more than you can imagine. I know that no matter how much I love you, I alone can't save you from addiction. You have to want it for yourself. You have to save yourself." Matthew just stared at me without speaking. I left and cried and prayed to exhaustion. I didn't want him to die not believing in God.

Not everyone believes in rock bottom, but I do. I think that a person has to be so far into his addiction that he sees no way out. You can check your child or loved one into rehabilitation, but if he isn't ready, the efforts will serve no purpose. You are wasting your energy and your money. In the Celebrate Recovery family support group, so many parents shared how they had lost their life savings putting their children through rehab only to watch the children go straight back to drugs. One parent even said their daughter stopped on the way home from rehab and got drugs. It cost them $40,000 to put her through a rehab program only for her to stop on the way home for a high. She wasn't ready. Some parents put their children through ten, twelve, and even more drug treatments centers. I listened to these stories in disbelief because I couldn't even imagine my husband paying for one rehab stint, much less ten. I figured that none of those kids had hit rock bottom and they were not ready to get well.

Effects On Marriage

JIM IS A GOOD HUSBAND and a good father, but he has very little patience for what he calls "stupidity." When he grew up he was a parent pleaser. He never did anything without considering whether his parents would approve. Even after we were married, before we made any important decisions, he considered whether his parents would approve. It was borderline ridiculous to me, but it was normal to him. To say that Jim didn't understand Matthew's addiction is no understatement. Over and over, Jim asked, "Why doesn't he just stop?"

At one point, I wasn't sure my marriage could survive Matthew's addiction. My heart was broken, not only by Matthew's words that he would never be back, but also by the fear of not knowing where my marriage was headed. So, I stopped sharing any information about Matthew with Jim. We didn't talk about our son during the worst days of my life. Jim wasn't interested in hearing about Matthew's drug use and he wasn't interested in hearing if I was enabling or giving him money. I don't think he would have cared that I let Matthew stay in an empty apartment, but I know he would have been mad if he had known I was giving Matthew money.

I know that men are supposed to lead their families and spouses should communicate, but I had no time to process any of that. My son was falling apart and detaching from his family. I couldn't let him walk out of my life. I couldn't let my husband push him out of my life. I knew I couldn't choose between the two of them, so I figured out a way to make it work. I handled Matthew's issues on my own. Again, guilt raised its ugly head. I felt so guilty. Guilty that I felt anger toward my husband. Guilty for feeling I had let my son down by allowing him to be pushed out of our home. Guilty because I could not fix Matthew's problem. I tried so hard to understand where Jim's heart was in all of this. I knew my marriage was worth saving. I knew he loved me and all of our children. I had to tell myself that he was handling this the best way he could. The problem was he just didn't know how to handle it. This gave me something else to pray about. I was exhausted. I felt so alone. I was broken but I knew God could fix what was broken. Jim never asked about Matthew. I never volunteered information. I was willing to travel to hell by myself if that was what it took for Matthew to get well. I was good at keeping everything from Jim. Looking back, I realize I was a great secret keeper, even in my marriage, which I cherished because I had so much practice from covering up the ugliness in my childhood home.

Parenting Other Children

I HAD TWO DAUGHTERS AT HOME who needed me but, because I was consumed with Matthew and his addiction, I felt like a neglectful mother, which, of course, compounded my guilt.

Courtney and Kimberly, fortunately, took up a lot of my time. I knew it was important to be there for them, especially at their ages: teen and preteen. They were always involved in some type of dance, gymnastics, or competitive cheerleading. I was constantly driving them to and from practices and competitions. That was good. We got to spend normal, healthy, family time together. I was forced to focus on them, which gave me reprieve. We had some really good times, which are now wonderful memories for us.

There were certainly days when I was pre-occupied. I was probably on edge and snapped too easily. I didn't discuss Matthew's problems with Courtney and Kimberly. I wanted them to love their brother for who he really was and not think of him in terms of drug addiction turmoil. They knew he loved them, but he had distanced himself from the family.

I never wanted Courtney and Kimberly to feel they mattered less than Matthew, but it's hard for a mother to balance her time and efforts when she has one child who is in trouble or has a greater need. I was extremely intentional in how (and how often) I cared for my daughters. I didn't want them to resent Matthew for taking up too much time.

Between my job, which took up many hours a day, and worrying about Matthew, there were days I was probably short with my daughters. When I hurt their feelings, I made a conscious effort to apologize.

I toggled between two existences. My mind was occupied at night, in the darkness, with thoughts of Matthew. I wondered if he was okay. I wondered if he was alive. In the light I worked to please a husband and two daughters who needed me. I tried to hide my anguish and exhaustion the best I could, but it was difficult. I constantly asked myself, *Am I being a good wife? Am I being a good mother?*

Even though I spent most of my childhood hiding my feelings and hiding my father's alcoholism, hiding my turmoil over Matthew was harder. I resented my father but accepted the situation. Matthew's problem was something totally different. He was my child. I couldn't talk to my husband. I couldn't talk to the girls. I wasn't ready to talk to most of my friends about it. Thank goodness, I had Jamie. With my father, I kept secrets outside the family, but with Matthew's addiction, I had to keep secrets *within* the family.

Financial Burdens

MATTHEW COULD NOT AFFORD ADDICTION. He stole and pawned things to get money to buy heroin. He had almost no personal items and lived a barren life. One night in the apartment, after taking a shower, Matthew came out of the bathroom to find two guys stealing his television. He owed them money, and they were there to collect. I am pretty sure that television was one of the many items I bought back from a pawn shop.

Matthew's drug addiction became my addiction. My life was consumed with worry and financial wrangling to keep him out of jail. I bought back all his pawned stuff. I paid off people from whom he stole. I covered his bills. At my house, I tried to hide anything of value because I knew if he came over, he would take anything he could pawn. The cycle was endless and I contributed to it.

According to the drug and alcohol treatment center The Recovery Village, the following are average annual costs of various addictions:

*Alcohol - $3,000+ per year.
*Marijuana - $5,000+ per year.
*Prescription pills - $32,850+ per year if bought on the street. OxyContin falls into this category.
*Heroin - $18,250+ per year.

Once an addict needs more and more Oxys to get and stay high, he typically switches to heroin because heroin is so much less expensive. Today, there is a whole new deadly addition to the problem; a lot of heroin is laced with fentanyl. Fentanyl in very small doses can kill.

People who do not have money and have no way to get money often participate in illegal activities in order to get the money for drugs. Acquiring drugs is a 24/7 job. Addicts "borrow" money from family members and friends. They know that as long as they are addicted, they will never repay the money. Some use their cars as collateral for loans and their cars end up repossessed. Addicts steal anything, from anybody, anywhere to support their habits.

Addicts may lose their family's support. Addicts may lose their children. It takes a lot of work and time to get your family to trust you again and to get your children back if they have been taken from you.

Rehabilitation centers can be very expensive. If you are lucky, insurance will cover rehab. Many rehab centers offer financial aid. Inpatient rehab programs can cost between $6,000 and $60,000, depending on the length of stay. Some rehab centers calculate fees on sliding scales based on length of stay and ability to pay. Some are free, but those are usually state-run and have long waiting lists. Because heroin is so lethal, heroin addicts are often moved to the tops of waiting lists.

My Isaac

THE DARKEST OF THE DAYS in Matthew's addiction were also my darkest days. The Beast was winning and I was losing my grip on everyone who mattered—my son, my daughters, my husband, and myself. I prayed constantly, but I was so scared that God wasn't listening or wasn't going to answer my prayers with the outcome I desperately wanted.

Isaiah 43:1 (ESV) reads, "Fear not, for I have redeemed you; I have called you by name, you are Mine." In this verse and many others, God commands us not to fear. When our children are young, we fear they will get hurt. We worry about their grades. We fear they will be easily influenced. We fear they won't make good choices. We fear they will be bullied. Parents fear that our children may be abused or abducted. As they get older, we fear our children will speed or text while driving. We fear they will drink, or worse, abuse drugs.

Finally, I had to ask myself the trite but crucial question I knew Matthew would eventually have to answer, "Are you sick and tired of being sick and tired?" I knew I couldn't go on. I had hit rock bottom when I had hoped he would hit his. I knew I had to crawl out of the hole and do whatever I could to go on, with or without Matthew. I had to ask myself the question that the lady at the recovery center had asked me when I called to make an appointment for Matthew, "Why are you working so much harder at saving your son than he is?"

A lot of addicts must hit rock bottom before they seek restoration. In the Bible there are several stories in which God allows people to hit rock bottom. God is not only the rock at the bottom, but he is also the foundation on which rebuilding a life must begin.

Letting go doesn't mean you don't care anymore, or you don't love your child. That couldn't be further from the truth. It's because I love Matthew that I had to let go. I did not want to be the person (enabler) who stood in the way of Matthew's hitting rock bottom. I finally realized I was killing him by enabling him to stay in his addiction.

One night, I prayed and prayed, and I am talking down on my knees, crying and wailing and begging God to help me stop personally battling The Beast because I just couldn't do it anymore, and I knew my efforts were futile. While I had always prayed for God to handle Matthew's life, I really just partially handed him over at night and kept taking him back to try to fix him the next day. I really had never *totally* turned Matthew over because I thought I should be able to take care of my child. I beat myself up so many times because I had failed. I was his mother, I knew him better than anyone—or so I thought.

Matthew didn't want to be a drug addict, but he thought there was no way out. I, too, was beginning to believe that was true. Death would be better than a life mired in the depths of addiction. I prayed a prayer that no mother ever wants to pray. I told God I would get out of his way. I promised to stop my enabling efforts to help my son. I knew that I was going to have to turn my back on Matthew even if it meant he might die. I let go.

The next time Matthew called to ask me for money was the last time I helped him. He said he owed some guys money and if he didn't pay him, they were going to kill him. I met him and gave him the money. I stood in that parking lot, looked The Beast in the eyes and searched those eyes for my son's soul. I somehow said to Matthew, "You need to listen carefully, believe what I say, and understand. I will not be giving you any more money. If you chose to not pay bills in order to do drugs from this point on, the consequences will be yours. Please don't come back to me with another excuse or threaten that someone is going to kill you. That is unfair, and I can't trust you. You are killing yourself, and I won't be a part of it any longer. I will pray for you every day. I love you more than you will ever realize. I am strong enough to do this and I mean it. If you ask for money, I will tell you, 'I love you, but 'No.'" I stopped giving him money, but it hit me that I had to stop lying for him. I had to stop covering for him. Was it scary to let go? Of course, it was. It was the hardest thing I have ever done.

I stood by my words and gave him no financial support, but I was still codependent in private. Instead of spending money, I spent time praying. I could turn my back on the drugs and behavior, but I could never turn my back on my child. I resolved to love him through his drug abuse.

God asked Abraham to sacrifice his son Isaac as an offering. Abraham never questioned or argued with God. Abraham didn't try to "fix" it; he just did as God asked. The night I prayed for God's help and let go to trust Him, I did the same. I laid down my Isaac, my Matthew. I gave him up to God. I had endured broken, stressful, erratic sleep patterns for years, but that night I slept all night long without waking up. I slept more soundly than I had in years. The next morning I woke up and I felt such a relief. The weight of the world was off my shoulders. A few days later Matthew hit his own rock bottom.

Missed High: *Matthew Explains*

I DON'T REALLY REMEMBER MY LAST HIGH or that weekend very well. I knew that I was in trouble. To use the term *support system* is a stretch, but the people I used on a daily basis, my support system, had run out. Whether they were my parents, my family, my friends, the people I used drugs with, and even people I didn't like, none of them would let me around them. I could take advantage of no one anymore. At that point I had stolen from, lied to, or cheated basically every contact I had. I could feel the walls closing in on me. Drug dealers wouldn't even take my calls. I needed a time out.

Someone I knew was actually going to treatment that weekend. He gave me about one gram of heroin on Friday. I was like, *Well, this is all I've got until however long.* At that point I had no intention of going to treatment. I just knew I had about a day's worth of heroin to use. I started using it. Half a day went by, and I was well ahead of the schedule that I had set for myself.

There's China white heroin, which is powder form. Then there's what's referred to as black tar heroin, which is the brown form. The amount you do depends on your tolerance. When I started using heroin, I probably bought half a gram at a time and was able to shoot that in two sittings. That's probably no more than twenty dollars' worth. That's why other drugs eventually lead people to heroin. Heroin is less expensive and more powerful. When I was buying OxyContin off the street, I would pay like 50 or 60 dollars for a single pill and shoot all of that at once. The first time I did it, I snorted a quarter of a 40 milligram pill, and it made me sick. I threw up half a dozen times. Why did I do it? I don't really know the real answer, but I think because my friends were doing it.

When you inject heroin, probably about three seconds go by before you can feel it coming on. It's not instant, but it's pretty quick. It takes the full three to five seconds before you feel it really hit you.

The drawback to heroin is that it wears off quickly so you start to get sick fast. Every day, pretty much as soon as the drug works its way out of your system, you start to go through withdrawals, but there is a process to it. The symptoms are very, very mild when they begin. First, you might yawn a lot. Your eyes water, you start getting sniffles, and your nose runs. Those are warnings and you know what is coming. After that, your body starts to hurt. You get cramps, your stomach aches, and you can't take fluid or food because you get bad diarrhea. Whatever you ingest, a minute later it comes out. Then, more body cramps come and your back hurts really badly. The worst part is not being able to sleep. All you can do is lie there and think of how miserable you are and how much pain you are in. That's just the physical part and less than half of the real suffering. There's a constant voice. The drug starts speaking to you. The *addiction itself* talks to you and says, "We have to do something about this."

So you're running through all these scenarios in your head and you know that whatever could make you feel better is just outside. If you can just get enough money together or get somebody on the phone who can get you drugs, all the pain will go away. That's the most difficult part. I've done it. I've thought, *If I can just figure out a way to throw a big enough tantrum, maybe I can con somebody—my mom, Jamie, whoever it is— out of some money, or I can steal something and pawn it.* It's a battle that never ceases. There's never a moment where you just resign yourself and say, "I'm going to get through this."

You steal from your own mother, your sister, your girlfriend, or innocent people that you don't know. This stuff feels bad. You can't deny it. You can trick yourself into not thinking you're an addict for a long time, but there's no way around it. Eventually, you can't hide from it, so you start to look in the mirror and believe all these things. You start to feel a certain way about yourself. You finally believe, "This is me. I'm a horrible person."

I knew I was an addict about the time heroin became a financially unsustainable habit. I didn't make a ton of money back then. I was working 40 hours a week and making ten or eleven dollars an hour. Friends and I would get together on Friday or Saturday. We might drink a few beers and buy a few pills. We tried a whole lot of substances until we really started to zone in on opiates. Once I did Oxycontin the first time, even though I threw up after, I'm somehow sure that I did no other drug again for a very long time.

Instead of using only on the weekends, I started carrying over the drug use to Mondays and Tuesdays. Then I'd start up on Thursdays. I got to the point where I spent my entire paycheck on opiates. I think there's actually a definition somewhere, like you're an addict when you start to do things that are outside of social norms or things that are outright illegal. You have negative consequences but you continue anyway. I would say that's a pretty accurate description because you start to realize that you don't really have control. I had thoughts like, *I can't stop. I need to not use all of my paycheck. Now I'm getting my paycheck on Friday and it's gone on Monday and that's the only thing I used it for. Now I have an issue. I don't have gas to get to work.* I would fill my gas tank up on Friday because I figured my money would be gone by Monday. Then I had to figure out how I was going to eat.

I heard a guy say one time, there's a difference between substance abuse and addiction. He used alcohol. He said if drinking starts to interfere with your work, you have a drinking problem, and if work starts to interfere with your drinking, you're an alcoholic.

Not long after I started budgeting to support my drug use, I actually lost that job and I started to bounce back and forth between employers. I couldn't go to work Monday through Friday because my paycheck was gone on Tuesday or Wednesday and I was sick on Thursday and Friday. I couldn't spend eight hours working because I had to leave and try to figure out a way to score something.

That wasn't easy. You start to meet people, but they aren't all connected. When you find a dealer, you don't want to share him with anybody. As time goes on, you expand your networks as widely as you can. Only when people are desperate do they share information. I've been all over the city, from really nice homes to houses and apartments that I didn't think I'd ever set foot in.

The first time that I did heroin here in Knoxville, the guy who was setting it up didn't have a ride. I picked him up and took him to a gas station. Sitting there in this gas station in the parking lot, I saw a Jeep Wrangler and I recognized the driver. He was somebody I knew from high school. He comes from a very respectable family, but he became a pretty serious drug dealer. I cut out that connection. I drove the Knoxville guy a couple times to a record store in Nashville to pick up. On the way there he was counting thousands of dollars on the dashboard of my car. On the way back I was nervous about driving with thousands of dollars' worth of heroin in my car. That would have been a wrap. I mean, I would have been done. Even just driving, I'm sure I would have been in prison for that. I know the dealer eventually went to prison.

I've heard Mom say that she saw me in the apartment stairwell and I stared through her like I hated her. I don't doubt that because I couldn't stand seeing her. I hated talking to her. It's exhausting to try to use people. The smarter they get, the more that they learn, the better you have to be at it, the more words you have to use, and the more effort you have to put into excuses. Then, if it doesn't work because they're on to you, it's totally frustrating.

Obviously, it's all incredibly selfish behavior, but it's like, "You can help me right now. Why won't you help me?" It becomes painful because you know that these people want you to take some accountability, and they want you to stop what you're doing. I didn't want to stop. That wasn't an option for me.

For the same reasons, I didn't go to church. Why would I want to be around anyone like that? I resented everyone. If you weren't dealing with what I was dealing with or weren't going to help me, I had zero use for you.

The drug culture is dangerous, but I was never afraid. There were times where I was certainly uncomfortable. There's no need to tell all of the stories, but I can remember one time when I was sitting in a parking lot with some drug connection guy. We were there to meet somebody we had been introduced to through a third-party whom neither of us knew. We were sitting across the street from a grocery store and waiting. Whoever we were supposed to meet was late. I looked in my side mirror and saw a police car pull up right behind me and block me in. I looked over at the guy I was with, and he reached into his jacket and pulled a gun out.

I remember thinking, *You have got to be kidding me. He's about to get me killed.* I asked him, "What are you going to do? Jump out of the car and start shooting?" It was a SWAT team. Within minutes, there were three or four police cars in the parking lot. He took the gun out and stuck it under the seat. I don't know that God intervenes in a moment like that, but the police pulled us out of the car and questioned us quite a bit, but they never looked under the seat.

Even a moment like that wasn't enough to stop me. I walked into houses where I saw pretty intimidating things, but that voice told me to do whatever I had to do. The only fear I had was of not being able to get drugs.

Mom's term *The Beast* is absolutely accurate. It may sound like a cop-out to some people, I think, but if you really understand what it feels like to be addicted, controlled, it makes sense. There's a song called "The Package" by the band The Perfect Circle. It's a slow melodic song told from the perspective of the voice that's in the singer's head. It's so insightful as the voice sings, "I'll nod and watch your lips move if you need me to pretend," and, "Then I'm out of the door again." As the song progresses, the voice gets angry and starts screaming and demanding. That really is what it feels like.

With a friend, my mom, or Jamie, I was very pleasant in the beginning and said everything that I thought they needed to hear. When that didn't work, I got more and more desperate. The voice gets louder inside of you.

Jamie was a good kid. She was a good girl. She saw things that she should never have seen. I feel like I've stolen innocence and purity from people in my life. That's hard to deal with. I absolutely brought pain on my parents that they should not have had to deal with. It's my fault. They didn't deserve that.

The voice, the addiction, made me say things that I wish I had never said to people and do things I wish I had never done. I'm not sure there's anything I wouldn't have done had I continued using because I did do things I said I'd never do. My conscience was absent.

When I would go into drug houses, for the longest time, for years, I could always look around and be like, *At least I'm not as bad as that guy or that girl.* As time went by, there were fewer people that I could say that about. It wasn't long before I was that guy.

I would lie down every night and say, "Please God, take this away from me. I don't want to be like this. I'm not doing this again tomorrow." I admitted it to Him every single time and I felt bad. Then I'd wake up the next day and start to get sick. It was like, *Okay, I have to do this. I need this one more time because I don't have another plan yet. Let me try . . . .*

Why in the world would God do what I asked? I was really just saying, "Will you keep me from getting sick, lying, stealing, and hurting people?" If I could just get high and not have any repercussions from it, then that would have been great. I would have gone back out and done it again the next day. That's not how He works.

Then it's like you need more of the substance to cover up the shame because once you put a needle in your arm, a lot of that stuff—the shame and pain that you feel because of things you've done and people you've hurt—goes away. The heroin numbs you, at least for a few hours. I always felt remorseful at night. I'd repeat, "Okay, I'm not doing that again." There's no breaking the cycle. I hated myself every day.

I always recall and appreciate how it felt to sit in my apartment that night. I was in a living room with a couch and a La-Z-Boy chair and not much else, other than drug paraphernalia. There was an entertainment center against the wall but there was no TV or PlayStation in it. I'd already pawned all of those things. I sat in that apartment all day long with nothing. I can remember and will never forget how lonely, how desperate I was. I used more heroin that day than I ever had in a single day. Late that night, I put a needle in my arm and I knew that I was pressing my luck. I knew that my plan to make this draw out was probably gone. I was like, "Well, this is more than I've ever done. This might be enough to kill me." *Hopelessness* is probably a pretty good adjective because I didn't really care if the heroin killed me or not. That night, I wrote a poem.

The Darkness

I live in total darkness
Because I cannot see the light.
I have everything to lose
And still can't put up a fight.
All I do is take,
Because I have nothing left to give.
I think I'm still alive
But have forgotten how to live.
Every night I fall asleep,
But I never go to bed.
I've woken up for 25 years,
But the last 4, I've been dead.
It's funny that they call it "Getting high."
That's strange; I've never felt so low.
I hold on so tight to something that isn't there.
Why? Just let go.
Still I live in total darkness.
Is there anyone here but me?
Will someone please open my eyes,
And show me how to see . . . .

Hope, Mystery, Faith

WHEN JAMIE KNOCKED ON THE DOOR to take Matthew to the drug rehab center, he opened it and didn't argue. He knew he had to go. He became agitated on the way there because it was an hour and a half drive, and he needed drugs. Even after he got there, Jamie wasn't sure he would stay because he was desperate to get high. Jamie left him. Neither of us knew whether he would stay or walk out.

Four days after Jamie had dropped Matthew off, I was in my office at home. I cried and prayed and asked God to help Matthew and me. I had no idea if Matthew had stayed at the treatment center. I had no idea if he was dead or alive. No one had heard from him.

While I was praying, I sobbed and asked God, "I don't know what to do. What do I do?"

God said, "Call." It was a clear voice in my head. God was speaking to me. This was on a Thursday at about 10:30 in the morning. Immediately, I phoned the center and spoke with a lady at the front desk. I told her my son had checked in there on Monday, and I just needed to know if he was still there. She said there was no way she could give me that information. I begged her to let me know, but again she said she was not legally allowed to give me any information on any patient. I started crying and told her I wasn't asking for any medical disclosure, I just wanted to know if my son was still there. She asked me his name. When I said, "Matthew Seals," she repeated his name loudly enough for anyone near her desk to hear her.

Then, I heard a familiar voice. "If that's my mom, tell her I'm doing fine." HE WAS STANDING AT HER DESK AT THE VERY MOMENT I CALLED!

That second, I knew that when God may seem the most absent, He is the most present. He is in the middle of circumstances whether or not you recognize Him. He spoke to me in the midst of my crisis. I became still. I knew that God was with my child and me.

God Worked On Me

GOD ANSWERED MY PRAYERS. God started healing me. I got stronger in my faith every day and stronger in my capacity to deal with Matthew.

It is SO important to remember that you shouldn't ENable an addict but you should BE-**able** them. Be able to support them, not financially, but emotionally and spiritually. There is a difference between enabling and supporting.

I do believe that one of the most important things we have to do is to love addicts through addiction no matter what. That doesn't mean giving in to demands or guilt. It means to tell them you have hope, and that you love them no matter what. They need *hope*. They need to know someone *cares*. They need to know they *can* get well.

They need to hear and be reminded that they do have options. When they are ready to make a change, they can. They haven't done anything bad enough that they can't be forgiven.

Matthew needed to be encouraged and not discouraged. He already felt enough pain to want to hide and be artificially soothed by addiction, both physically and emotionally. I get so angry when I read comments from people on websites when they say drug addicts are scum of the earth, that they deserve to die, etc. If we encouraged addicts more, they might find some self-worth. Matthew couldn't have felt much lower than he already did. Being consumed by addiction was like being in the bottom of a deep, dark well with no ladder and no rope. He saw no way out. As loved ones, we can't enable, but we can throw addicts spiritual ropes of love, encouragement, and prayer instead of shaming them back down into that well to die. It is possible to climb out with the right kinds of help.

One More Day: *Matthew Continues*

I DIDN'T INTEND TO KILL MYSELF; I would never say that. I don't even know that I had the guts to do that. I just wasn't afraid of dying. With that last high, I just thought, *Well, I'll try it. I'm out of options.* I knew I was in trouble. I had done bad things and knew I was about to pay the consequences. I was probably going to jail. I just thought, *Well, I'll either go out with a bang or this will be the end of it.* When I pushed the plunger down, I remember thinking, *Wow. This may be a bad thing.* That's the last I remember.

When I came to, I was confused and didn't know what had happened. It was daylight. I had a journal and had written a bunch of odd stuff in it. It was there on the couch. When I woke up, I thought, *Oh, my God.* My arm was all swollen, and I wasn't really sure why. I don't think I ever got the needle out of my arm. I think it probably was in there all night. Instead of thinking, *Man, I almost just killed myself,* my reaction was, *I can't believe I just wasted all those drugs and missed my high.* It was a very visceral reaction, that anybody, any addict, would have had because you don't want to waste any drugs.

I think that most addicts are trying to walk the line between killing themselves and getting high because most of the time, you're not getting high anymore; you're just fighting off the sickness. You just scrape enough together to avoid getting sick.

I went to treatment only because I didn't have another choice. I had no one. I had nowhere else to go. I'd done some form of detox half a dozen times, and I had called that treatment center and made appointments to go, but I never went. I didn't have any serious intention then. At least once or twice I used that as leverage, like, "If you'll give me a hundred bucks or whatever just to get me through then I'll sign up and I'll go." There's usually a waiting list of a week or two. When that day would come, I would find a reason not to go.

That morning, I was physically out. I didn't have any more drugs. My entire existence at that point was just a constant daily grind to try to find drugs. I was empty. I was out of options.

People I'd stolen from were threatening to press charges against me. I just thought, *Here's my motivation for going to treatment.* This is the honest to God truth. I thought, *Okay, I'll go. I'll stay for 30 days and let all this stuff die down. Everybody will think that I'm doing better. The people that are talking about pressing charges will let it slide because I went to rehab.* It was just a preservation thing. I needed a time out.

If I told you that I got in the car that day and rode with Jamie to treatment because I wanted to change my life, I would be lying. One hundred percent. That first day that I got there the voice talked louder and louder. When I arrived, I asked for a medication that helps you go through withdrawals. They wouldn't give it to me. They didn't even have it there. I said, "I can't stay here then," and I told them I wanted to leave.

That is was how irrational I was. I was saying that I was taking my bag and leaving. But if I walked out onto the street in Johnson City, Tennessee, I had no one to come pick me up. I genuinely didn't think that Jamie or my mom would. I was close to doing it.

Then this girl came up to me. I had met her through the years. I had seen her sick before. She said, "I know how you're feeling." She'd been there probably a week at that point. She said, "You don't want to go out there. You can do this. Just give it a day or two."

I remember looking at her and thinking, *If you can do it, surely, I can make it through one day.* I knew I needed to stay because if I walked out, I was alone. If I stayed 30 days, the pressure would fade. I thought, *Okay, but I can't stay on my own.* That moment, I was like, *All right, need some help here.*

Outside the rehab facility, you could smoke or play basketball or walk around. Once you're in the program, if you go outside you have to have a staff member with you. But, you have free will. You can walk off, but close to the sidewalk there's a line. You can't go past that line. I walked up to that line, looked up, and saw a church a block away. That's probably the first time that I prayed something different than, "All right, God. I need you to take this away from me." Instead, I prayed, "I need you to keep me here for another hour." Then, I prayed, "I need you to keep me here another three hours." Then, "Another day, another three days, another week."

As time passed, that was my go-to. I also did a lot of processing and small group therapy.

Once you're in rehab for a while, the fog starts to lift a little bit and you laugh again. You smile. You have fun. You come back to life. If you take a picture of people the day they walk into rehab and the day they walk out, they look physically different. After a couple weeks people around you start to say, "You seem like a good guy. What are you doing in here?" One day you're able to look in the mirror and think, *Okay, maybe I'm not this horrible person. I don't have to be this horrible person. I can be something else.* Maybe that's the person that Jamie always saw.

I've spent numerous years dealing with stuff and making amends to people. I've talked about my addiction fairly openly for a long time. It's funny. I almost take offense when every once in a while I'll share my past with people their reactions will be like, "Wow. I would never have thought that in a million years." They tell me what they pictured my life story might've been. That's good. If I ever told my story and someone reacted, "Yes, I can see that," that would *not* be good.

I do remember the first time that I ever held a narcotic in my hand after I was clean. I was a nursing student and doing my clinical rotations at a medical center. There was a patient in there who was getting liquid Dilaudid, which was actually one of the drugs that I used to inject. The nurse said to me, "Go in the med room and grab the two milligram vial."

I said, "Okay. Well, what do I do with it? The patient was only ordered one milligram. What do I do with the other milligram?"

She said, "We just throw it in the bio-hazard container and we waste it."

I went in the med room by myself. I pulled the patient's milligram into a syringe. I held the vial in my hand and I looked at the leftover one milligram of liquid Dilaudid. I thought, *I could take this home and I could use it, and nobody would ever know.*

Right then, I processed through the moment. I thought, *You know what? No one would ever know. That's the bad part because I wouldn't get caught. I'd get away with it. Maybe I wouldn't be back the next day to rob the place, but a week later, two weeks later, a month later, I'd do it again. Then, I'd do it again, and then I'd do it again.* Eventually, someone would've come to work and their medication machine would've been empty of narcotics, because I'd have taken all of them.

It feels good to be high on heroin. It's the best feeling I've ever felt. There's no way my words can do it justice. It was fake, though, because I wasn't really there to experience the high. If you watch someone high on heroin, you'll see that he's just nodding out and barely conscious. And when I wasn't high, I was miserable.

Somebody said to me one time, "Everybody can get off drugs. Everyone who leaves the detox program has gotten off drugs. It's learning to live without them that's the hard part." If you get high again after you leave detox or rehab, the only reason is because you wanted to get high more than you wanted to stay sober. You have to start figuring out why you shouldn't get high. You have to build a case.

I used to tell people when they would leave a 30-day program, "Go for eight days without using. If life isn't better, if your life doesn't improve, then just get high again. Just wait eight days and see. I bet you'll have a little bit more money. You'll have some freedom, some choice. You'll sleep. You don't actually have to do what this thing inside of you is telling you to do all the time. You can become a free human again. You have to start making a list."

As the years have passed, I have added more to my list: my great relationship with my parents and sisters, my wife, my children, my career. If that evil voice in my head starts to come back to life to trick me again, all I have to do is remember that I'm one decision, one milligram away from self-destruction.

If I did heroin today, it would probably make me sick if it didn't kill me. I also believe I would very much love the high all over again. That's just honest, and it frightens me. As long as I believe that, I won't do it even one time to find out because I know where I will end up.

Before, when I was sitting in that empty apartment by myself, I didn't have much to lose. Now, I've come a long way. I'm married. I'm a father. I have a home. I help people. I'm not proud to be a drug addict, but I am proud to be one who is recovering.

A Much Different Experience: Jim

TO ILLUSTRATE HOW DIFFERENTLY FATHERS may address a child's addiction, I asked Jim to share his experience firsthand. These are his words:

I had no idea Brenda was riding up and down the roads looking for Matthew. I never knew any of what she was doing and never even suspected it was happening. The normalcy in our home with our two daughters was uninterrupted. Brenda had this dual, split life, so to speak. I don't know how she pulled it off. Naturally, I would think that if you are dealing with this, wallowing in the mud in one part of your existence, and putting on a face of normalcy in the other, life would be very difficult. In front of friends and associates, that would be hard, but at home it had to be even harder. We didn't sit around and talk about it. We didn't wonder what we should do, or any of that.

I don't know if some of it was based on the fact that I'm Matthew's stepfather and Brenda is his genetic mother. Maybe she thought, *This is my cross to bear and I'm going to deal with it*, even though Matthew has been my son since he was seven years old.

Maybe she knew that I'm not emotional about a lot of things. I take more of a common sense, rational approach. We would certainly differ in how we handled Matthew's problems. In retrospect, I was too rigid, but it was just so nonsensical to me. The whole subject of addiction is one of insanity. I just couldn't understand *why*. I couldn't wrap my mind around why someone would do it. My empathy toward addicts is much better now.

When it was brought into our home and going on and on, I finally said that I was done. All of the macerations relating to it caused me to finally say, "Enough." I made Matthew leave. The whole drug culture is disgusting as was his second detox attempt at our house.

Fathers and mothers are different. My dad always said that if a kid robs a bank, the mother will hide him in the basement, but the dad will call the police. There's some truth to that. My enabling threshold was lower than Brenda's. If I had been involved from the beginning, I would have pulled the plug long before she did, but maybe to the detriment of Matthew.

She had to be exhausted, but she's a machine. At the time we had a pretty significant apartment business, and she ran all of that. I've always said that one day her head's going to fall off, and these wires are going to come danglingly out. She pulled it off. She did it somehow. I've always marveled at her strength. Brenda took that burden on all by herself. Maybe she just wanted to have normalcy in some part of her life—our house. As a kid she had this normal life at school and with friends, and then she went home and dealt with the demon of her father's alcoholism. People compartmentalize; maybe that's how Brenda got through it. She wanted to make our house a safe place.

Brenda could have opened up to me, but that might have caused problems. My opinions would have been different from hers, which would have caused friction between us. If we had started arguing about this on a daily basis, there would have been so many conflicts. Parents have different ideas about lots of things, but Matthew's situation was catastrophic, so we likely would have encountered all sorts of disagreements. Brenda shielded the rest of us from the ugly part of addiction. Brenda kept the drug culture from coming into our daily lives. I don't know if that was good or bad. I don't know how she did it, but she did. Her taking on all of this kept our marriage and our daughters' home intact.

Looking back, I've learned a lot about how to deal with addiction. Parents think they can cure addiction, and they can't. The sooner that we stop the enabling, the better. From a parent's standpoint, all you can do is tell a kid that you love him and that he has a future with opportunities. I do think that's something important that helped Matthew. He knew in the back of his mind that if he could get past addiction, there were opportunities for him. I mean, we were saying, "Here's an education. Just pick it up. Just go do it." Some kids aren't as fortunate, particularly, those with no financial backstop, no way to get an education, or no family support. Plus, many have arrests and convictions that prevent them from getting jobs. They may think their lives are in the toilet anyway, so what's the motivation to stop using drugs? Matthew knew his life didn't have to be in the toilet.

Everything I've learned about drug addiction, I learned from Brenda. Parents should, number one, make sure children know that they love them, number two, not enable them, and number three, show children they have opportunities and a future beyond addiction.

I also learned that it can happen to anyone, regardless of socioeconomics, home life, or personality. Matthew was a likable kid. He wasn't a daredevil. So, you wonder, *How can this be?*

Most kids go through a stupid phase. You can define that any number of ways. My grandmother called it "fool's hill." She would say, "If you can just get your kids over fool's hill, they'll be fine." For kids, it comes down to a lack of maturity.

I remember telling Matthew, Courtney, and Kimberly, "The only reason you would try drugs is that you think you might like them, but the worst thing that can happen is that you do *like* drugs. Now what are you going to do? It's insanity. Don't try it." I can see someone falling into alcoholism because those beverages are everywhere, but with any addiction, once you are physically clean, why in the hell would you go through it again? There's something in the brain, some craving, some weakness. I don't understand it, but obviously there's a huge drive pushing you to use the substance again and again. Why pick up a gun with two chambers and put it to your head when you know one of the chambers holds a bullet? With drugs, people are picking up the gun.

I always thought, *There is NO way any of my kids will ever do drugs.* You think you are doing everything reasonably right, and assume addiction won't happen, but most kids are going to go through the stupid phase; you just have to hope it's not drug use.

Don't assume that doing all of the right things as a parent will help you to bypass this issue. Parents need to be diligent. Education and fear are probably the best motivators. Kids in high school may not respond to being rational. They hear and absorb education. They respond to fear. The threat of rehab or seeing a before and after picture of a meth addict may work while talking may not. Kids aren't genetically stupid, they are genetically immature, so they do stupid things. We just have to get them over fool's hill. Parents have to bob and weave through all of the minefields of immaturity.

I still worry a little bit about Matthew. Maybe *worry* isn't the word. Addiction is a subject that I still don't understand as well as I should. I don't want to *have* to understand it anymore. I know that if things happen in his life, he likely has a fallback position. As a parent, I can't help but think, *He did it once. Would he do it again?* There are certain times when people hold their demons in check, whether those are psychiatric problems, alcoholism, bad habits, etc., but as you get older, you start fraying at the edges. You can't always hold everything in the boundaries. Sometimes people veer off if things get bad enough for them. Some people are mentally tougher than others. How do we deal with life when things go south?

Matthew's addiction is way in the back of my mind, but it's there. We never talk about it. There's no need. What good would come of it? What's the point? "Let's talk about when you were young and did something stupid. Let's talk about all that hell we went through." He's in a healthy situation, so there's no good in rehashing. If he falls back into it, we'll talk about it, of course. In the meantime, why get all exhausted and anxious about it? It helps our relationship that we can be together without me being judgmental and damaging his self-esteem. He has overcome addiction and created a wonderful family and life. He's a good solid guy.

Maybe some parents have endured so much, they can't let go. Maybe parents like that just need reassurance from the child, or maybe some parents harbor resentment for all of the heartache and loss the child's addiction has caused. I don't resent Matthew for the hell he put Brenda through. She could, but she doesn't. In the grand scheme of things, the money, the time lost, and the school issues are insignificant compared to his being healthy. Brenda and I are very proud of Matthew. Everything is good now.

Of all the scenarios that could have played out, ours couldn't have played out better, thanks to luck, God, Brenda's perseverance, and Matthew's efforts.

Courtney

MATTHEW WAS JUST THE BEST big brother. I know this sounds cliché, but it's true. He is nine years older than I am, so you'd think he wouldn't want his little sister around, but he always let me hang out with him and his friends. I liked to sit in his room and watch them play video games. He was always so cool and I looked up to him. He even let me ride around and listen to music with him in his car. He was an awesome brother. I guess I was about nine or ten when he moved out, but he'd still visit with me. He made me feel loved. He was dating Jamie, and Jamie is like a sister to me.

I remember the night that he came home and Mom found out about his drug problem. He had been at the movies. It's hard to remember the details, but I remember he came into my room and lay down on my bed and just cried and cried. He gave me a huge hug and hugged me for a long time and said he was sorry. I was in shock because he had never acted like he was a drug user to me.

I was so young that I attributed drugs to people who lived on the street. I didn't know how to handle the news that Matthew had a problem. I did ask Mom questions, but Mom and Dad never said much about it. I was in the dark until I got a little older. I wondered how he was doing. He would come around here and there, but he wasn't the same. I was really confused. I still loved him. For those few years, I remember I just missed him so much.

When he tried to detox at home, he was so sick. I wanted to help him but didn't really know what to do. I wanted him to feel better. I would hang out with him for a little bit, but there were times when he was really sick. It was strange. I felt helpless. I missed my brother and the way that we used to be. I didn't know the extent of his addiction until years later when he was beginning to get well.

I got the sense that he was embarrassed and ashamed of himself. Now that I'm older, that's how I explain it. He wouldn't joke around. He wasn't outgoing. I didn't want him to feel bad physically or emotionally. I worried about him, especially when there were long periods of time when I didn't see him.

During that time Mom was still there for my sister and me. She did everything she always did, but I could tell she was stressed. There were a lot of late nights when she was up worrying, talking with Jamie, and tense. There seemed to be a lot of phone conversations about Matthew, always behind closed doors. Mom had an office in the house; it wasn't uncommon for her to be awake at three or four in the morning, and she would get up with us at seven o'clock and go all day. There was no change in how she cared for my sister and me. We were super active and constantly needing her. She was able to carry on. She never faltered in taking care of our whole family. Looking back, I don't know how she did that.

I went to a fine high school, and there were drugs all around me. I was most exposed to drugs from around age sixteen to twenty. I saw cocaine, mushrooms, ecstasy, all kinds of stuff. Usually, drugs were at concerts and music shows. The users were the children of my parents' friends. It wasn't like I was running around with a bunch of gang members.

My parents didn't really talk about drugs when we were little. If it came up in conversation, they would just say, "Don't do drugs." There was never really a conversation; there was just an understanding that our parents didn't want us to do drugs. I think parents make a mistake by assuming their children won't see drugs. They should have the conversation and prepare children on what to say and *how* to say, "No." My good high school girlfriends knew some about Matthew. I had no desire to try drugs because I knew that I could try something one time and become addicted.

Through all of this, one of the bigger things I think I've learned is that drug addiction, or any type of addiction, can affect literally anybody. I hear all the time, "Oh, he's just a drug addict. We should just get rid of those types of people," and stuff like that. I grew up with my brother, and he is an amazing person. He has a great family. He just happened to get involved in something. He didn't want to go down that road. The road took hold of him. Everyone has demons, and no matter how successful someone is, he has issues, and this can happen to anybody. I think Jamie and Mom helped Matthew tremendously in overcoming his addiction. Jamie stood by him the whole time. It's amazing. I think if she had left, it could have turned out a lot differently. You have to love people through their problems with tough love, but you have to let them know you love them no matter what.

I don't think about it much these days, but I know Matthew has a lot on his plate. He has a young family, he works hard, and he gets stressed like everyone else, but I hope he has coping mechanisms that are healthy. I worry a little. I guess that's always going to be there.

About my mother . . . I learned that my mom is a rock star. Now that I'm older, I can appreciate her more. I assumed every mom was that good, but they are not. She's like a machine. I can't believe her strength. She's been through so much in her life that I'm just in awe of her. I don't know how anyone could go through what she's been through and be the mom and woman that she is. I know motherhood is exceptionally difficult, especially when you go through difficulties like hers.

I remember my parents arguing, normal stuff, but now that I know all that went on, I think it's awesome how their marriage stayed strong. Now, they are closer than ever.

Seeing Matthew with his kids lightens everything. He's a great dad. When I think about where Matthew was and where he is now, I'm so proud of him.

Kimberly

I WAS YOUNG when Matthew went through his addiction, and my parents kept me pretty sheltered from it so there isn't a whole lot I remember. I am not sure exactly how old I was when his battle with addiction really started, but the first memory of it was when I was in the sixth grade. I was in the computer room (his room) working with my friend on our science fair project one night. At that point my brother wasn't living at home anymore. I remember hearing the side door downstairs slam shut and someone running up the back stairs and into my mom's office. At that point I could hear a lot of yelling and crying between Mom, Dad, and Matthew, and I started to get an idea of what was going on. I remember feeling scared, disappointed, and embarrassed. I told my friend to go home, and I listened in on some of their conversation through the door. What I remember most was my mom crying a lot, my dad doing more of the yelling/questioning in disappointment, and my brother also crying and saying he was sorry over and over again. I went to bed pretty confident that I understood what was going on, but I never had the guts to ask anyone about it.

It wasn't until Matthew went to the Army that I understood for sure. While he was away at basic training, I got a letter in the mail. My brother and I weren't super close growing up. He was always a great brother, and I looked up to him and thought he was so "cool," but being twelve years younger, it's not like we ever ran in the same crowd or had any of the same hobbies or anything like that. That being said, when I got this letter I was really taken by surprise. It was a couple of pages long, but, basically, he told me what he had been going through and how sorry he was that he hadn't been a better role model. He told me how proud he was of me and how much he loved me. He also promised me that he would get better. I remember crying and reading it over and over again and feeling really hopeful.

Like I said, my parents kept me in the dark about Matthew's addiction, and I'm glad they did. I was too young to be exposed to all of that, and I know they didn't want me to look at Matthew differently. They wanted me to enjoy being a kid, and I'm very appreciative.

For me, the worst part about Matthew's addiction was seeing my mom and dad hurting. I could tell it was just absolutely tearing my mom to pieces, and even though I know she tried to be strong for my sister and me and put on a front, she was just absolutely falling apart. She cried a lot, mostly at night. Looking back, I wish I could have been there for her, but she was so busy being a bad ass mom that she tried to never let her pain show in front of me. I never truly knew how awful it was until I was older, and she felt like I was ready to know.

As terrible as that time in his life was, in a strange way it influenced me by making me want to stay away from drugs and all of that mess. I saw the way it affected my parents, Jamie, and Matthew, and I just knew I never wanted to get caught up in it. Now that Matthew is on the other side of things and THANKFULLY has earned a happy ending, I could not be prouder of him. I am extremely grateful that he has not only beaten his addiction, but he has also become an amazing husband, brother, son, father, and Christian. I look up to him in so many ways, and I love him more than he'll ever know.

Jamie

WE WERE TOTALLY IN LOVE. I was living in Spain temporarily. At the time, my communication with Matt was limited to weekly e-mails and payphone calls. Our conversations were always positive and uplifting. We were constantly professing our love for each other, sending each other poems and song lyrics (Matt's a fantastic writer), and telling each other how much we missed one another.

We couldn't wait to be together again. It was all very sweet and romantic, except for this one phone conversation. I remember standing outside at a payphone in the middle of downtown Madrid. I was taking a minute to give Matt a quick call before going out with my friends. I don't remember his exact words, but Matt was sad and crying and telling me how he didn't deserve me, that he wasn't a good person and so on, but he was vague and didn't get into any specific reasons for why he felt that way.

I never thought for a second that it was anything serious, I just thought maybe he was feeling insecure and missing me. It was in December and I had been gone for almost five months, so I did my best to comfort and encourage him by reminding him of my love for him, of God's love for him, and of the great man he truly is. I didn't think about that conversation again until after my return home when he later told me he was struggling with addiction. Then the call made sense.

After returning home from Spain, Matt and I reunited, got engaged, and quickly started planning our wedding. I was still living at home with my parents, and Matt was on his own. We were happy, but after a couple of months, I realized something was off, not with our feelings toward one another, but in Matt's disposition. He was staying up really late, sleeping in late, rarely had any money, and was getting past due notices for bills.

For a while I thought it was just a result of living next door to good friends. He spent most of his time with them. I thought they were just getting caught up playing video games all night and living the "typical" college lifestyle. I continued to gently press him by expressing my concern that something was off, that I was worried about him, and that whenever he was ready to talk, I was ready to listen. His attitude remained positive, not at all defensive, which is surprising considering the secret he hid.

Finally, one night he said to me, hesitantly, "I'm addicted to pain pills." I was shocked. I don't know what I expected, certainly not that, but I was relieved to know the truth and proud of him for telling me. I quickly realized how hard that must have been for him and wanted him to feel safe and know that he could trust me to love him, unconditionally. I wasn't at all angry. I was thankful to know the truth. What a terrible secret to keep and how guilty he must have felt. I didn't want to make him feel worse. Instead, I wanted to help him through it by showing him love, forgiveness, and compassion.

I told him something like, "We'll get through this. Whatever we need to do, we'll do. Please don't worry. You can do this, especially with God; everything is possible. I still love you." At that moment, he and I were hopeful. I think he was relieved, as was I, but we had no idea the challenges and darkness we'd soon face. We were both so young and naive, but my innocence, along with our love for each other and God's powerful hand, are what kept me hoping for so long.

I had no experience with addiction personally or with anyone else, so I had no idea what to do. I was naive to think it would be easier than it was. It was an emotional journey. Matt made several attempts to detox and stay sober, with the support of his family, of course, but without any consistent counseling or making any real changes to his lifestyle, other than not using, his attempts were short-lived and unsuccessful. Each time he'd relapse quickly, and the signs that he was using again were obvious. Through it all, I struggled, too. It was so hard watching him lose himself to his addiction. It was the hardest "thing" I've ever endured. I wanted to fix him so badly, more than anything. I prayed nonstop. I cried a lot. I didn't tell anyone, although several friends already knew and hadn't told me. I found out later that a few close friends had pressed Matt to tell me. If he hadn't, they would have.

His mom and I struggled through it together. I leaned on her. We kept each other up-to-date and spent endless hours on the phone listening to and supporting one another. It often seemed like when one of us was feeling weak, the other was there to provide strength. I'm so thankful I had her during that time.

Matt's addiction definitely challenged our relationship. When he was sober, we were fine, but when he was using, it was torture. My love for him never swayed. I knew his actions were a result of his addiction, and I also knew I couldn't be with him if he was using. He knew it, too. But throughout his addiction, my focus wasn't on keeping us together. It was on keeping him alive, out of jail, and, this may sound cheesy, but about pulling him back into the light. I felt my purpose was to "love him through it," "to be a light in the dark," and, most importantly, to remind him he wasn't alone—no matter how alone he felt. Eventually, I reached out to get help through Celebrate Recovery for myself and for Matt. We went through tough times, the toughest, but I ALWAYS believed God's grace and powerful love could change Matt's heart and make him "new" again, which is why I never gave up on him, always forgave him, didn't take his addiction personally, and did my best to see past the sin that was controlling him. Instead, I focused on the beautiful man inside Matt, whom I loved so dearly.

Credible, Accountable

FINALLY, I SAW MY SON when, several weeks after he entered the treatment center, I was allowed to visit. Remembering how horrific his detox attempt was at my house, I asked him how he managed to stay at the center. He explained the line at the end of the property, and the center's rule that if you crossed that line, you were out of the program. He told me how on that first day he stood there sick, sad, lonely, and ashamed. He contemplated crossing the line. Agonized, he looked up to see a church a couple of blocks away, the sun shining on its steeple. He asked God to help him stay one more day. He did that every day for the first week.

In the rehab center, patients had to get on their knees at night and put their shoes under their beds. They had to also get on their knees in the morning to get their shoes out. Matthew later told me that during those times, he prayed. I know the counselors encouraged it. Matthew finished the program and came home detoxed and clean.

After Matthew got clean, he told me, "Mom, if you had kept doing what you were doing, I would have kept doing what I was doing." He confirmed what Celebrate Recovery had taught me. I wasn't responsible for his addiction, but my giving him money and lying for him helped Matthew stay in addiction.

Several months after he finished treatment, Matthew was at Celebrate Recovery. He was going to give a general talk, but not tell his personal story. The group's leader, Gil, stopped Matthew right before he went on stage. He told Matthew that someone in the room needed to hear the truth. Matthew froze. On the way up to the podium, he asked God to give him the words. He didn't even speak the words he had prepared to say. He let God talk through him, and he told his addiction story.

A couple of days later, the church received an envelope in the mail and in it was a napkin. The person who wrote on the napkin said something to the effect that he didn't know why he stopped in Celebrate Recovery that night. He wrote that a young man was on the stage telling his story that night, and that story matched his own. He said he used drugs, but after listening to Matthew and their shared experience, he said to himself, "I will not use drugs tonight." Gil gave the napkin to Matthew the next week at the Celebrate Recovery meeting. I don't know what happened to the guy. He must have done well enough to put the note into an envelope and send it to the church, so maybe he didn't use the next day either. I hope he was able to get clean. You never know what effect your story will have on someone else. You never know what others need to hear, but it might be exactly what you have to share. Tell your story over and over.

A New Foundation

ABOUT NINE MONTHS after Matthew came back from treatment, the apartment building that I owned and where Matthew was living burned down. Matthew lost everything and had no insurance. I was on vacation and he called me to tell me he was watching the building burn. He was calm, but I started crying. He asked me why I was crying and I said, "Because you lost everything."

He said, "I have more than enough." He told me that the fire department asked everyone in the building if they could get one thing from each person's apartment, what should the fireman get. Matthew told them he wanted his Life Recovery Bible and his pictures. They were able to save both for him. Matthew said the rest was just "stuff."

Once the building was cleared of the debris, I found myself standing on the foundation that had survived the fire. I remember thinking that I would rebuild the apartments on that foundation. Then the thought occurred to me that that a rebuilding had already happened. If the fire had happened a year before, it would have been a reason for Matthew to go get high, but that year, with God's mercy and grace, Matthew was building a new foundation and God was rebuilding my child's life.

What Can A Mother Do?

I HAVE LEARNED A LIFETIME of lessons during Matthew's addiction and recovery. Looking back, I am better able to see my mistakes and Matthew's vulnerabilities. We are all searching for happiness and contentment. I believe everyone is born with a God-sized hole that they search and search to fill with material possessions, obsessions, or addictions. Matthew was at a vulnerable time in his life when young people start searching for their personal contentment and happiness. We think, *If I own this, I will be happy. If I had a better job, I would be happy. If my parents didn't fight, I would be happy. If I had a girlfriend/boyfriend, I would be happy.*

I've often heard that The Beast targets people who are weak. I believe Satan targets people *when* they are weak. We are all weak at times. As parents, we must teach our children that they can't always avoid failure or weak moments. We must teach them how to face those moments so that The Beast has no access.

The Beast tries to convince his target to fill emptiness with earthly pleasures. We can never be satisfied by drugs or material things. I call that emptiness, that hole, the "Jesus hole." I believe if you fill that hole with Jesus, you will become "whole."

I'm by no means an expert in relationships, addiction, therapy, or Christianity. I am a flawed human who has the capacity to learn and evolve.

What works? As I stated before, there is no one-size-fits-all solution. What works for one person might not work for everyone. I totally stand behind Celebrate Recovery because I know it worked for me and for my son. I have seen it work for hundreds more.

There are studies that support treating opioid addictions by using other medications such as Suboxone or Methadone, but many people do not believe a person is really clean if he uses one drug to stave off another. Using medications to reduce cravings or avoid relapses can offer hope and reduce the emotional and financial costs of substance abuse. You should check on the pros and cons of all medication-assisted treatments and do what you think is best. Hopefully, if the choice is to used medication-assisted treatments, the addict will eventually get off those medications.

Some people suggest interventions. I am not sure how I feel about interventions and have never been involved in one, but if you think it will work for your child or loved one, it's worth a try, but only with a professional interventionist.

The right treatment center may be hard to find, choose, or afford. Don't give up. You need to not only check out their success rates, but also speak with someone who may have been through them. One way to do that is attend some type of family support group or a recovery program in your city and ask for recommendations. Just because a facility costs more doesn't mean it is more effective. There are some facilities that are partially or entirely subsidized by the government. More and more insurance companies are including rehab in their policies as they understand addiction is a treatable condition.

Relapsing is not uncommon, so don't be totally discouraged if the addict relapses shortly after treatment. Hopefully, the addict will get back on track and stay clean. If the addict has the tools to get clean and stay clean, it can work.

Information is a powerful tool. If you have a loved one who is addicted to painkillers or heroin, read everything you can. Get counseling for yourself, too. I can't emphasize enough that even if your addicted loved one won't go to rehab, you need to attend a family support group or a codependents' support group. You must educate and protect yourself.

You must also protect your marriage and/or family. Men tend to work out their emotions looking for solutions. Women like to express their feelings outwardly through tears and body language. We like to talk through our problems or share our feelings.

Jim wanted to solve the problem by telling Matthew to just stop. I am so happy that Jim and Matthew are now close.

YOU. CAN'T. FIX. EVERYTHING. I have sat in family support groups and listened time after time to parents who are exhausting themselves as they try to fix their adult children. I've known parents who do their kids' homework, do their school projects, do their book reports, take children things they have left at home just to keep them from getting bad grades. I have done all those things. If kids don't learn how to fail when they are young, they will not handle failure very well as an adult.

Parents can help their children by being loving and strong. It starts with simple conversation. Young people need to be exposed over and over and over and over to the ramifications of drug abuse. They need to see pictures of meth users. They need people to go to the schools and talk to them. Parents, be nosy and trust your instincts. If you suspect your child is using drugs, have him tested. Be in the room when he takes the test. Better yet, take the child somewhere and have a professional test him. I have heard parents ask, "What can you do when they are fifteen and sixteen years old?"

My answer might be, "Does your child live with you? If so, you have total control. Take away privileges, car keys, bedroom doors. Set boundaries and stick to them."

Healing is possible. If you have never had a relationship with God, it doesn't make you a bad person, and it certainly doesn't mean you can't be made whole or be healed.

We are all sinners. None of us are better than anyone else. Even Christians get it wrong. The meaning of brokenness is ruptured, torn, not functioning properly, weakened in strength, bankrupt. According to this, we are all broken at times. I had to wonder how long Matthew would be broken or if he would ever turn his life around. Psalm 34:18 (NIV) reads, "The Lord is close to the broken-hearted and saves those who are crushed in spirit." Matthew was broken, but not beyond repair.

Matthew wasn't the only person who recovered during this time. I found my way. I also found a purpose. I have always felt there was something I was supposed to be doing in my faith. I kept asking God if I should write this book and if He wanted me to, to please send signs. I saw signs everywhere. I pushed them away for a while, but God finally told me, "Be still and write." It has taken a long time to put this story into words. Even though Matthew has been clean for a long time, these pages were hard to write.

We often hear the cliché that God doesn't give us more than we can handle, I think God DOES give us more than we can handle. If He didn't, we would never turn to Him or ask for His help. Matthew 11:28 (NIV) says, "Come to me, all you who are weary and burdened, and I will give you rest." To me, He is saying that when we do have more than we can handle, we should come to Him. You can trust Him to carry your load. I've always thought I was very tough because I've endured so much in my life, but the time did come when I knew I needed help. I was weary and burdened and God gave me rest. He can do the same for you.

If you are an addict reading this book, I want you to know that you can get better! My son is proof that you can get well. He went from marijuana to OxyContin to heroin. Who knows what else he may have taken? I never asked and, at this point, I don't really want to know. I do know he was the sickest I have ever seen him. There were so many demons. The Beast was always with him. The good news is, the Beast and the demons can be dealt with. There is a better way of life, but you have to be sick and tired of being sick and tired. You have to remember that you have been sick for a long time and it will take a long time to get well. Don't give up. You are loved! Take it one day at a time.

You have people who love you and want you to get well; even people you don't even know are praying for you. Every breath you take is a new beginning. Addiction isn't a death sentence. It is treatable. Millions of recovering addicts have gone on to live fully productive drug-free lives. We must understand and love people who are suffering in addiction.

In that spirit I wrote this upside-down poem.

Son Down, Son Up

Drug addicts are not good people
So don't try to tell me
That they are worth saving
Because we all know
They are worthless, awful people
And nothing will make me think
They deserve to be loved
Realizing they are someone's child and
That the pain might be too hard to bear
Makes matters worse, and just
Because we say it could happen to anyone
We have to ask, why do we care?

Now, read the poem again, but from the bottom up.

I was asked to be on Knoxville, Tennessee, radio station Joy 620's show, "Drive at Five." Host Jenny Bushkell and I discussed Matthew's addiction. I told Jenny and her audience about the night I hit rock bottom. I explained how I finally realized I couldn't help Matthew and had to give Matthew over to God and trust and be obedient to God, just like Abraham did. When I left the radio station, I got a text message from Matthew. I didn't know he was even listening to the interview. My child's message read, "Way to go, Abraham."

Today

MATTHEW HAS BEEN CLEAN now for fourteen years. I don't know how Jamie stayed with Matthew during the darkest of times, but I am so thankful she did. If she had been my daughter, I would probably have told her to not walk but run away. I admire her and give her thanks and praise for staying by his side. I'm not sure what Matthew would have done, or if he would have gotten through the dark times without her. They've been married for thirteen years and they have one son and one daughter. Matthew returned to college and graduated with a Bachelor of Science. He is now a well-respected supervisor.

No one wants to imagine a child or loved one becoming addicted to drugs. That happens to other people, right? When you hear that someone's child is addicted, you start wondering why: Was he a troubled child? Was there an underlying problem? What caused the addiction?

Some people become addicted through prescription drugs when they are hospitalized or recuperating from an injury. Some get addicted when they try drugs recreationally. No one says, "Please give me a pill because I want to become an addict and ruin my life." You do not have to be a bad person to become addicted to drugs.

The negative perception of people who become addicted to pills needs to change. The Beast wants to rip apart families. It looks for the least, the last, and the lost. We need to look for them, too, and help them.

As I wrote this book, I realized three things that could come from my work. The most important is to bring hope and to assure readers that they or a loved one can overcome drug addiction. The second is to make parents or loved ones understand they didn't cause the addiction, and they cannot stop it or cure someone. The third is to call attention to the fact that good people can become addicted to drugs. The shaming and name calling must stop.

When I read that a "celebrity" has overdosed, the comments people write are heartbreaking. Addicts are sons, brothers, husbands, fathers, daughters, sisters, wives, and mothers. Why would anyone give up everything for nothing?

I hope Matthew will never forget his rock bottom. I hope he never forgets the chains that bound and imprisoned him. I hope he never forgets the price of those chains and what it cost him at the time. I know I won't.

I still don't know why my son took the first pill. I do know that God's love is greater than any control The Beast can muster. Matthew is now a light in a dark world. The Beast took my son down into his darkness. God brought my son up into the light. Matthew was not alone, and neither was I. As far down as my son was, God helped my son up.

To the Beast,

You tried your best to take away my son like you have taken so many other sons, husbands, fathers, mothers, daughters, sisters, and loved ones. While I raised my son and loved him for eighteen years, it took you giving him only one pill to turn him into someone we didn't recognize. You steal the souls of the addicts and then you go after their loved one's souls. While I don't know why my son invited you into his life in the first place, I thank God he was finally able to find the strength to turn away from you. Some addicts aren't so lucky and constantly struggle. For those, I pray that they will be able to one day walk away.

You are a master of deceit. You make people do things they would never normally do. You make addicts lie, cheat, and steal for you. You turn them into manipulators. You make them turn away from their friends and families—unless you can convince them to bring everyone along. You make them feel good in the beginning but like crap at the end. You make them sick and tired. You even make them willing to die for you daily. They are willing to lose everything for you even when they have so much to live for. I know you have no heart and you certainly have no feelings and no soul.

But, I know there is Someone more powerful than you. You can be defeated. You can be destroyed. I only hope that my book will reach someone, anyone, who will tell you, "no."

Sincerely,
A mom who never gave up hope!

Acknowledgments

I am extremely grateful to so many people for encouraging me to write my story and not giving up on me even when I kept setting it down. Without your support, I would have never finished *Son Down, Son Up*.

Thanks to Rita Wooten, one of my prayer warriors and best friends, for praying and encouraging me to tell my story—knowing it was worth sharing. You have been there for me during good times and bad, always listening and offering support. Through your belief in this story, you led me to my publisher, Jody Dyer.

Many thanks to Terri Gianeselli for being the first person I turned to, outside of my family, when I found out about Matthew's addiction. You were instrumental in my seeking help from Celebrate Recovery.

To Jody Dyer, my editor and publisher, thank you. I began with literally hundreds of Post-it notes and notebook pages on which I had written thoughts and stories. I was lost and not sure how to even start. Even when I repeated my thoughts and stories, you were always patient and understanding. You led me in the right direction, got me started, and walked with me every step of the way.

I cannot express enough my appreciation to Dr. Gil Smith, Celebrate Recovery minister, for always being there to listen and provide emotional and spiritual support. I felt like I had nowhere to turn but Celebrate Recovery may have saved my sanity. I look forward to the day you put your story in print.

To my daughter-in-law Jamie, I am so thankful for your being there with me and for me during such a difficult time. You have an amazing faith and a lot of patience.

My family has been behind this book from the beginning. Jim, you have been one of my biggest fans. Thank you for your patience and support. Kimberly, Courtney, and Matthew, you have expressed how proud of me you are for writing the story and that makes me smile on the inside. Thanks to all of you—for adding your own contributions to this book. As a parent you wonder if you are doing the right thing and raising your children in the right way. I know now I must have done something right. You all make me so proud. Love you more!

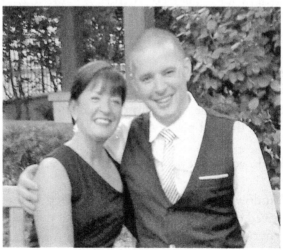

Brenda and Matthew

Discussion Questions

1. What do you think about Brenda's choices for the title and subtitle of the book?

2. How does the book change your idea about the drug culture?

3. How did specific passages or poems affect you?

4. How does Brenda make readers more aware of and knowledgeable about different issues related to addiction?

5. How did your opinions of Brenda, Jim, Matthew, Jamie, and other family members change over the course of the story?

6. What do you think Brenda did right? Wrong?

7. Where do people, especially children and teenagers, get drugs in the first place?

8. Why do you think people start taking or abusing drugs?

9. What do you think is the best way to keep your children or loved ones from *trying* drugs? Do you think they listen to the old slogan, "Just say no?"

10. How do you think you would feel if your found out your child was using drugs?

11. How do you think you would react? What changes in behavior would you make, regarding affection, communication, financial support, prayer, and so on?

12. If your loved became an addict, do you think you would be an enabler or a supporter?

13. How do you think you would fight the urge to be an enabler?

14. How would you emotionally cope while your child or loved one was suffering? Would you be ashamed and keep the addiction secret, or would you tell friends and family? What kind of help would you seek?

15. Do you think your family would be supportive or would they want to kick the addict out of the home?

16. How would having a child addicted to drugs affect your relationships with other family members and friends?

17. Would you be willing to turn your child over to God, no matter the consequences, or would you try to "fix" the situation yourself?

18. Would both parents be on the same page or would you have a conflict? How would you deal with it if your spouse wanted to handle it differently?

19. How can families safeguard belongings, money, heirlooms and trust while trying to help an addict (before and after rehab)?

20. How can friends and families keep addicts engaged in normal life activities?

21. What are the different ways loved ones can seek personal help while a friend or relative is immersed in addiction?

22. If someone you know is addicted to drugs, what do you have in common with Brenda? How do you differ? What did you learn from Brenda that can help you cope?

23. There is great difference of opinions on whether addiction is a disease or a choice. What do you think?

24. How do you feel about mandatory prison sentences for drug dealers and drug abusers who get caught?

25. How involved should schools be in drug education?

26. How should school administrators, counselors, and teachers help a child whose parent is an addict?

27. What do you think governments, churches, law enforcement, and healthcare providers can or should do differently to help addicts?

28. Did the book succeed in accomplishing what it set out to do, which was offer hope to those who have a loved one or friend in an addiction?

29. Why would you suggest this book to someone else? Who may benefit from reading Brenda's story?

Made in the USA
Monee, IL
29 May 2020